Healthcare Under Duress

Healthcare Under Duress

An Inside Look at the University of Washington Billing Scandal

Swannee Rivers

iUniverse, Inc.

New York Lincoln Shanghai

Healthcare Under Duress
An Inside Look at the University of Washington Billing Scandal

iUniverse, Inc.

For information address:
iUniverse, Inc.
2021 Pine Lake Road, Suite 100
Lincoln, NE 68512
www.iuniverse.com

ISBN: 0-595-32008-2

Printed in the United States of America

I would like to dedicate this book to my family. First, I must thank my husband, James, for his continual support and encouragement during the many hours I spent reliving this emotional journey to complete the book. Also, to my baby chicks: Patrice and Paris. My oldest daughter Patrice, aka "Mom's number one cheerleader," thanks for all the times you were willing to entertain your sister so Mom could write. Paris, my "little one," I want to thank you for the humor you always manage to bring into my day. Thank you all for the joy you add to my life.

Roxie, my dear friend and "adopted sister" in life, I must thank you for living the experience as a former UWP employee yourself and the understanding that you have offered me for so long. You are a one-of-a-kind woman.

Mark, I must also thank you for your continual reminders that there is such a thing as justice. Thank you for your willingness to put your life on hold and your determination to continue the fight to expose the truth at all costs.

Swannee Rivers

Contents

Introduction

Why write this book? I had to. Since the 1980s, when I first hired into and discovered evidence of illegal billing within the University Physicians (UWP) organization, I knew something had to be done. As a former thirteen-year employee, I maintained a vast array of positions within the company: Medicare Abstractor, Medicaid Abstractor, Commercial Abstractor (Aetna, Blue Cross…), Support Coordinator (abstractor and assistant financial counselor), outpatient medicine clinic coder, assistant cardiac catherization biller. These positions allowed me to obtain expertise in the medical billing field as well as to gather a clear understanding of the business processes within the company.

However, despite my changing work positions through the years, the level of deception continuously elevated. I continued to maintain hope that one day others would learn the truth about these practices. Perhaps I could somehow bring about a change.

Too many questions remained unanswered. Why were so many individuals within a well-respected organization willing to look the other way in the face of injustice? I wanted the public to understand that for years some have fought for change. Why didn't anyone seem to know? Others just wanted more insight into UWP's organization. I was able to provide answers. In the end, I needed to understand if there truly was such a thing as justice.

Swannee Rivers

Author's Notes

Some of the names in this book have been changed in order to maintain the dignity and privacy of others.

This book recounts the personal experiences of the author during her employment with the University Physicians and briefly post-resignation as she recalls them.

Thoughts of Yesterday

I sat at my desk with trembling hands and sweaty palms. Slowly, I began to massage the aching in my neck as I glanced at the date on my calendar. It read November 30, 1995. Forcing my body to remain almost motionless, I awaited the signal. A few minutes later, my private intercom buzzed. With the speed of a cheetah I lunged forward, nearly knocking the telephone over as I did.

Quickly whispering "hello" into the receiver, I waited.

The husky voice on the other end asked the million-dollar question: "Is it safe?"

Despite knowing I was the sole individual in the office at the moment, my inner fear forced me to look around. It was my co-worker Mark Erickson, wanting to copy some medical reports. As soon as the words "all clear" escaped my lips, the only sound remaining was a sharp *click!*

Sitting in my chair, I gave the receiver a tight squeeze and prayed he moved fast. His hurried footsteps echoed as he entered the office. Our eyes met briefly, but we did not speak a word. There was no time to talk. We each knew there was limited time to copy these reports that had missing medical documentation. Copies would be put into a secret folder Mark had created six months prior. What would be done with the reports later was not yet determined, but somehow we hoped they would come in handy. For now, this was a major step towards proving evidence of massive illegal billings that were occurring within University Hospital.

I watched as the lid to our office copier flew open and large piles of medical papers were thrust into its auto feed. Known for constantly jamming, I silently prayed this wouldn't be one of those days. Surprisingly, it accepted page after page. The copies could be seen gently falling into the tray on the right side. Everything was progressing smoothly. Within minutes, a familiar sound interrupted the activity, causing my eyes to bulge.

The sound of heels rapidly clicking on the hallway floor, playing a familiar tune jolted me—*rat ta tat, rat ta tat*—the noise was unmistakable. I would know that sound anywhere. I immediately gave two coughs as a warning signal. Mark grabbed his papers from the copier as quickly as he could, the print job was canceled, and everything was thrust inside the medical file. As he turned towards the door there was almost a collision, and I gasped.

Offering a polite "excuse me," Mark's attempted look at innocence was greeted with a stern look by our manager, Janine. Her face was anything but happy at that instant. Janine's behavior was unpredictable and the staff had become familiar with inquiring about her mood as the first task of each day. If you discovered that she wasn't happy, it was best to maintain a low profile until she felt better.

"Watch where you're going," she replied harshly. Placing one foot inside the office, her beady eyes darted back and forth suspiciously. Finding nothing to her satisfaction, she turned towards the hallway.

Inaudible mumbling was heard as she left, without saying a word to me or glancing in my direction. Feeling slightly relieved, I exhaled, but I knew there was trouble. Mark still needed time to get the photocopied papers put into his desk and it was up to me to offer a diversion, because sharing an office with Janine meant he was limited on what he was able to do at all times. Quickly grabbing a medical file and HCFA (Health Care Financial Agreement) form, I ran out the door as well, following Janine. Running across the hall I turned the knob, entering Janine's office seconds behind her. Feeling frightened, I noted the rapid pace of my heartbeat as I approached her. Talking to Janine always made me feel uncomfortable. She turned to face me, her face showing surprise. I began scrambling for words while struggling to maintain eye contact. This conversation had to appear convincing.

"I need help locating a particular report in this medical file. I have looked through the entire chart, but I can't find it. Would you mind helping me?" I managed to ramble off. Instantaneously, her face filled with her familiar look of irritation. I swallowed and forced myself to ignore it. This was one time I couldn't afford to let it intimidate me. Mark needed my help, even though he wasn't in a position to say anything to me at the moment. I held my breath and waited, silently praying she wouldn't ask me to leave and come back later. She glanced one last time in the direction of her desk, gave a deep sigh, and motioned for me to follow her into her cramped working quarters that was once a broom closet. The plain white brick walls made the room feel stifling. I walked in slowly, careful not to disturb the large pile of papers resting on her chair. The top of her desk was askew. It looked like a tornado had just passed through. I wondered how she ever managed to get any work done. Pulling a chair up next to hers, I opened the file and began talking before too much time lapsed and increased my discomfort level. Pulling a blue rubber finger from her desk and placing it over the top of her right index finger, Janine began frantically flipping through the pages of the chart in search of the operative report I needed. I had successfully captured her attention.

The sound of a file drawer closing in the distance caused me to glance over my left shoulder. Mark and I locked eyes briefly as he nodded to me, indicating that everything was put away. No evidence remained. Once again we had made a collection without anyone else discovering what the real mission was. This time we were almost caught, and that was a little too close for me. Turning back towards Janine, I exhaled and knew the next time would have to be planned differently.

Within minutes I understood why I wasn't able to locate the report I needed. It wasn't there. This situation was all too familiar. However, I had to admit I felt a sudden rush of relief flow through my body. The thought of having Janine locate the report made me tremble. If that had happened I would've been forced to sit through at least ten minutes of lecture about why I hadn't been able to find it myself. Of course the lecture would have been contained with some sort of sly insults. Through the years this had become a common tactic for Janine. Most of the employees had experienced this reality by now. I later came to understand that this was Janine's method of ensuring her superiority.

Janine flipped through the chart a second time and confirmed "It's not in here." Slamming the chart on her desk, she slid it towards me, barking out orders as she did so. "Go get a Request For Documentation Form" she continued. "Send it to Dr. Tolliver and tell him to document the report if he wants to get paid."

Why does she always have to use such a harsh tone? I wondered after a momentary hesitation I began to speak, unsure that I had heard her correctly. Explaining the procedure had occurred two years prior; I waited for new instructions, but was taken aback by her fierceness now.

"*So!*" She shouted towards me. The sound of Mark clearing his throat made us both turn in his direction. I knew he had done this to remind her that someone else was there. Somehow I knew this would make little difference.

I explained that I wasn't questioning her authority but was unsure if the physician would document for a procedure done so long ago. Somehow I felt she wasn't processing this information correctly internally, but her next response showed no signs of backing down.

"He'll do it; that's the way we have done it for years," she stressed. There was nothing left to say. I reluctantly gathered my paperwork and headed towards the door. My eyes brushed across Mark's face, attempting to gather his response, but it showed nothing.

"Thank you," I called over my shoulder. There was no response, because Janine had picked up the telephone receiver and was dialing a number. The room was quickly filled with the sound of her laughter.

"What are you wearing tonight?" I heard her ask. I wondered which friend she was chatting with this time.

That's all she ever thinks about, I thought as I left silently. Opening the drawer to my desk, I located the necessary form and filled it out, requesting documentation on this old procedure. What I was about to do made me very uncomfortable, but if I wanted to keep this job, it was necessary to follow company procedures. Stapling the upper left-hand corner of the paper and sliding the completed form into an envelope, I sealed it with a small strip of scotch tape. Tossing it onto the gray department cart we used to transport files to the Medical Records department, I wondered if I could get the necessary documentation. One week later my answer came. Delivered to me was the requested report with the *original date of procedure on it*. Glancing at the report, I wondered how a doctor could remember what he had done during a procedure on a patient two years prior. I attributed it to taking good notes. Stapling the report to the HCFA form, I was unaware how familiar this routine would become to the staff members.

"*What?*" Janine asked in a shrill pitch. There she stood at my co-worker's desk, hands resting on her hips and feet tapping repeatedly on the floor. My co-worker Megan Ross pulled back slightly. Megan and I had become co-workers earlier in the year when she was transferred from the University Physicians' main office on Eastlake Avenue due to carpal tunnel syndrome. She needed a position that wasn't as demanding on her wrists. Management felt the best position to place her in was that of an abstractor at University Hospital. Megan was a welcome addition from the beginning, and her fun-loving personality caused us to become instant friends. I found myself looking forward to our daily conversations on subjects that ranged from new dishes to cook, relationships, current events…Nothing was off limits, and we remained comfortable with whatever discussion developed.

Janine questioned Megan about a file she was working on. Beginning to stammer, Megan took a deep breath, starting her statement and began speaking softly. Her voice was barely audible. We had been friends long enough for me to realize that she was nervous. Janine had mastered the art of intimidating all those who surrounded her. I watched, slyly. Also, I was curious as to what the nature of the conversation was. It was then that I learned an operative report that was needed by the insurance company was located in the patient's chart, but Megan had encountered a problem. The documented report failed to contain the physician's required signature. This signature was required for our organization (University Physicians) to receive payment. Janine's frustration was visible, and appeared to be mounting by the minute.

"Those damn physicians!" she blurted out without so much as a glance around her. She appeared to be unconcerned about who might overhear this conversation. I continued listening, noting the bright red coloring in Megan's cheeks. I wished there was something I could do to help her, but past experiences within the department had made me aware that it was best to remain silent if the situation didn't involve you directly. I sat motionless, but felt a slight churning in my stomach.

Megan broke the momentary silence by asking what she should do. Janine argued that sending this particular report back would prove useless because of who the physician was. He wasn't quick to respond to documentation requests.

"I don't want you to send this back to the physician because it will take too long, and he probably will never sign it anyway," Janine snapped.

Janine instructed Megan to sign the physician's signature herself and forward the report on to the main office. I couldn't believe my ears and stifled a gasp. Standing next to Megan, with eyes blazing like daggers, Janine waited. I wondered what she would do.

Janine snapped at Megan, urging her to do what she had been told. Looking on, I bit my lip as my head hung in sorrow. I knew Megan didn't have the strength to say "no"; she was too frightened. At last Megan picked up the pen that was resting on her desk. I could see it tremble within her grasp. Slowly moving across the page, it finally came to a resting point. Appearing proud, I watched Janine as a smirk graced her lips.

As if reasoning with a child, I listened as Janine explained how simple that was. Before another word could be said, she turned towards the office door.

Her body moved seductively as her patent leather pumps made their familiar *rat ta tat, rat ta tat* sound. Only then did Megan and I allow our eyes to meet. We were both too frightened to speak, stunned by the transaction that had just occurred. Finally, Megan broke the silence.

Speaking barely above a whisper, Megan asked me if I had heard the transaction.

"I did," I replied, nodding my head. My eyes were enlarged. I felt them bulging. The lump in my throat almost prevented me from speaking. She pressed on, wanting to know if I had witnessed the entire transaction. I responded with a firm "yes."

Megan asked only one thing from me. She asked that I speak up for her and act as a witness if this situation ever came to light. Her words were chilling. "*I just forged a physicians signature.*"

"I know you did," I commented. There was nothing else to say.

As fresh tears dripped down her face, Megan explained to me how intimidated she felt; she felt trapped with no way out. It was something that didn't need explaining. I clearly understood. What she did was wrong, but at that moment there were no other options. Anyone who knew Janine would understand. Slowly raising my right hand as if taking an oath, I looked Megan in the eyes and made her a promise.

"If anyone ever asks about this day, I will speak the truth. Don't you worry." Wiping her cheeks with her hands, Megan began working again, as did I. Each of us vowed to never speak about this day again unless forced to.

My eyes moistened as I remembered the numerous days similar to the ones I have mentioned. There were too many to count. Opening the final drawer of my aluminum desk, I pulled another folder out and tossed it into the box beside my chair-a box that contained years of medical notes I used to perform my job on a daily basis. Lifting it in one swift movement, I had to adjust the box; it was heavier than expected. However, that didn't matter. I had everything I needed. Moving slowly towards the door, I hesitated momentarily. I needed to take one last look. Thirteen years of my work history, thirteen years of my life, and thirteen years filled with memories of co-workers I now called friends rested in a box. My tears flowed freely. There I stood, remembering how it all started and what had brought me to this day.

Discovering University Physicians

It seems like only yesterday. In 1982, as a recent high school graduate, I began preparing for college at the University of Washington. Through a mutual friend I met John Reed, vice president of University Physicians. He offered me a part-time position within the company after our first meeting. I wondered why, but I agreed to telephone a company manager, Loretta Wilkins, the following Monday. We spoke briefly and she invited me to interview for a current job opening. Arriving at her office located within the University Hospital—room D-207—her warmth immediately embraced me. Running her fingers through her salt-and-pepper colored hair, Loretta gently explained that this was just a formality. John had sung my praises. Without having a real interview, the words I had prayed for passed my ears. "The job is yours." Looking at her in awe, I readily accepted. I had just become an employee of the University of Washington Physicians *without an interview.*

My desk was located in room C-214, across the hall from Loretta's. Bagels, coffee, and juice were set on a nearby table and one by one, fifteen co-workers came to the small, neatly arranged office to welcome me. Stephen Jackson, a recently divorced father of one, and Sandra Nelson, a single, thirty something, free spirit, became my new office mates. I felt welcomed and accepted by all, as well as excited to learn the various aspects involved with processing medical claims.

Job training commenced immediately and I was soon introduced to two current books that would play important roles in my new job: *CPT (Current Procedural Terminology,)* and *ICD 9 (Internal Classification of Diseases.)* Using these books would help me learn the art of converting medical terms and procedures into numeric form, which in turn were processed by various insurance companies for payment. Stephen and Sandra made learning fun, and day-by-day I slowly began grasping concepts.

Loretta offered daily encouragement. From the beginning she advised me to pace myself, because "it will take about a year to learn everything." That provided relief, but her support only made me try harder. I wanted her to understand that I may have been "given" the job, but I was capable of doing it.

Six months later our department received some disturbing news. Loretta had made a major decision about her future, thus deciding it was time for retirement. We were all thrilled for her, but knew her absence would be a tremendous loss to the department. I wondered who would take her position. An answer arrived within days.

Louise Hines, a six-year UWP employee from the corporate office would take over. I had spoken with Louise on the telephone almost daily for the past year about patient accounts, but knew very little about her. She was a pleasant-sounding woman with an East Coast accent the size of Mount Rainier, making her voice unmistakable. Our conversations were consistently lighthearted, and I soon found myself relaxing about the impending change. The management transition occurred within a month. Saying our final goodbyes, we all waved frantically as Loretta descended down the hallway. Watching the disappearance of her silhouette, I sensed that no one could ever take her place.

An immediate change soon became evident within our department. The gentle, telephone persona I had associated with Louise fell by the wayside. A determined, aggressive, middle-aged woman emerged, seeking a rise in the corporate ladder at all costs, was revealed. The insensitivity she displayed was startling. She ruled the nest, and she made sure everyone knew it. No one dared step in her way. Our environment was changing rapidly, and I disliked what I saw happening.

Louise ran a tight ship, but she did a terrific job at keeping the department in quality condition. She was usually one of the first to arrive in the morning and often one of the last to leave. Employee favoritism became evident, but I wasn't as impacted by many of the complaints I heard from co-workers because I worked part-time. My focus was on my work, and I limited my involvement with office politics. I wasn't as happy as I had been working for Loretta, but things were manageable. I just hoped there wouldn't be too many more changes.

It had been almost two years since Louise had taken over. I knew my job well, and was proud of the success I had accomplished. As my fifteen co-workers piled in to our small office for a 9:00 am meeting Louise had called, I grabbed a legal tablet and prepared to take notes. My ears perked up once Louise began speaking in a soft tone. She was normally loud, so I sat at full alert. Something was different. Her behavior today was odd.

"You all are a wonderful group to manage, and I have enjoyed it tremendously," Louise began, "*but* I have accepted another position at the corporate office. I will be leaving this department at the end of this month."

Groaning was heard throughout the room. Louise raised her hand slightly, requesting silence and showing her appreciation for the obvious disappointment concerning her resignation. Gazing at my co-workers, I was startled by this unexpected, loud response. I was thrilled with this news. Today was a great day. I sat patiently waiting to see what else would come. It took all my strength to muster up a look of disappointment. Four years passed before I discovered a startling revelation: my co-workers sitting in the room with me that day were as thrilled as I was. They were merely too frightened to say otherwise.

Three weeks later a new transition cycle began for our employees at University Hospital. Louise needed to be replaced and the company wasted no time in making those preparations. Janine Turner, a five-year UWP employee and billing coordinator, was hired as the new manager. This decision surprised few. During the past two years, Janine, Louise, and another employee, Monica Parsons, had formed a friendship similar to a high school clique. Their private huddles, continual whispering, and smirks of joy they wore smugly upon their faces still remain as clear as a picturesque landscape in my mind. They acted superior to others, always, so I worried about Janine taking the reins. What would it mean for the rest of us once she acquired a position of authority? There were times when Janine was friendly, so remembering those times, I tried to convince myself things wouldn't be too bad. What choice did we have? Little did I know what was to come.

It wasn't long before more disappointing news passed my ears. My friend and office mate, Sandra, was moving on. She would continue working for UWP, but she had accepted a promotion to profee coordinator at Harborview Medical Center. I was shattered. Suddenly, all that had felt so comfortable and familiar was placed upon shaky ground. I didn't like it. During our final workdays as office mates, Sandra's whispers of "everything will be fine," did little to comfort my questionable internal feelings. Did I feel this way because it was my first *real job* and I had never experienced volatility in a work environment? I pulled myself together enough to give her many heartfelt congratulations. I truly was happy for her.

Janine takes the Reins

Megan Phelps was hired to replace Sandra. A rather shy, forty-something woman, I found her demeanor interesting when she first entered our office. She appeared to not really want to be there, and as I answered questions about the responsibilities of the job, she appeared frightened. I giggled as I found myself reciting the same words said to me when I started my job. "It will take you six months to a year to learn the job." That time estimate was accurate. Megan was transferred from the main office and I played an active role in her job training. The corporate office seemed to realize she would be a good fit for our department. The moment we met, I believed she would be, too.

Megan adapted well and Janine was extremely supportive during the first few weeks of her transitional phase. Megan asked many questions and found herself settling nicely into her new work environment. Janine remained approachable and helpful to Megan. As time passed, my observations noted the responsibilities of Janine's job mounting. She no longer managed her stress level well, and at times its ugliness began to show.

Janine had fallen into management with a vengeance. I was impressed with her drive. She was pleasant most times and when she had questions or needed added support from the staff, she asked. I felt guilty for the developing concerns I had regarding her. It wasn't fair; she was just trying to do her job. I hadn't given her a chance, or was it that not enough time had passed to confirm my suspicions?

My intercom buzzed, and glancing downward, I was surprised to see that it was Janine calling.

"Hello," I answered while scribbling down a quick note so I wouldn't lose my thought.

Janine requested that I come to her office.

"Sure, Janine, I will be right there." She hung up the telephone so quickly I wondered if she had even heard my response. Entering the cramped room, I gazed around, wondering how she could stand working in these tight quarters. I was already feeling claustrophobic.

"Sit down, please," she said, shuffling through some papers on her desk.

At last her hand rested on a manila folder which she pulled out, opened, and began flipping through. Handing me a paper, she indicated it was something she wanted me to work on. My expression must have been one of confusion, because I had no idea what she was talking about. The paper contained a long list of patient names and their hospital account numbers.

Her conversation began about an upcoming Medicare audit. I nodded, acknowledging that I was aware of this. In the past I had always heard the rumblings from my co-workers as audit time neared. It was a time when our office was filled with elevated tension levels. This wasn't merely because auditors were coming, but because of the pressure to ensure patient medical files were adequately documented prior to their arrival. This didn't impact me much because of my rotating work hours. I routinely missed a great deal of the "rush-rush" activity. But things were about to change.

Janine explained that this year there would be a change concerning our audit preparation. I listened, without saying anything. Her slight pause was an indication she hadn't finished her thought.

"I am going to involve you this year," Janine continued. I was surprised by this new information, but I welcomed the challenge. I was sure some of the gossip I had heard about audit time was exaggerated. "You have been here for a while now and have proven you are capable of assisting us and I think your help will be valuable." I smiled, appreciative of the rare instance of praise.

"Thank you, Janine." The last thing I needed to know was when to start these new responsibilities.

My new task was effective immediately. That was why I had been given the list of names. The list contained charts Janine wanted me to request that couldn't be obtained from Medical Records. I was instructed that if they were nowhere to be found in Medical Records I should locate them within the hospital. Janine made it sound so easy. The hospital was huge. There were eight different floors and numerous departmental wings on each one. *What about my other work?* I wondered. I only worked twenty hours a week. Somehow I knew there wouldn't be enough time for everything. Sensing my concern, she continued. Janine stressed that my first priority was *the list*. Any other job responsibilities I had were to be put on hold.

"Do you understand what I am saying?" she questioned without blinking. *"Nothing comes before this list."*

Yeah, I understand, I thought, *I am going to have a backlog.* Exiting her office, I felt my excitement dwindling slightly. With the list in my hand, I walked towards my office and couldn't help but wonder how she had gotten the list in the first place.

Re-entering my office, Megan and Stephen looked up in time to capture my concerned expression. In her usual gentle tone, Megan asked if everything was okay.

The words "No, not really" rolled from my lips rapidly. I continued to explain.

"I have just been asked to help locate some charts for the upcoming audit and was wondering how I would keep up with my other work." Glancing at me with a questioning look, the wrinkle in Stephen's brow indicated his understanding and showed his concern.

They each reminded me that I would have to do the same as everyone else: put everything to the side except what was pertinent to the audit. I would have to work on everything else as opportunity allowed. There was no other choice.

I reminded Stephen this was possible, as long as no one complained about my backlog. Returning to my seat, I pulled out medical record charge-out slips and began filling them out, requesting the needed files. It took forty-five minutes to request all the files on the list and by the time I finished, my right hand had a severe cramp. Megan had just departed for a lunch break and I knew it was the perfect opportunity to approach Stephen with my nagging question.

"Stephen, can you answer something for me?" I asked delicately. He turned towards me with piercing eyes and nodded.

"Why are we pulling files and checking for documentation *before* the auditors come? I thought they were coming to check the documentation for us, or is there something I don't understand?" I wanted answers.

Putting his index finger to his lips, I hesitated as he said "*Ssshhh.*" His face grimaced as he explained that this was a conversation we shouldn't have.

"What?" I pressed on. I wanted answers. He just shook his head as I stared.

Walking towards the office door, he removed the doorstop, allowing the door to close quietly. The sound of its *click* chilled me. What was so secretive that it required closing the door? As Stephen explained the audit scenario, I gasped in horror. I had just learned that the company was changing more than I realized and I wasn't sure I liked it.

Entrance into the World of Audits

My arms struggled to push our office cart, which was now loaded with medical files. The loud screeching of its wheels seemed to echo the sentiment my heart felt at that moment. These charts were pulled faster than expected, and as I strained to enter the cargo elevator I prayed the load wouldn't shift and spill once the doors closed. My mind was still reeling from the information I had just learned. Most companies didn't have the privilege of knowing when auditors were coming to investigate, but UWP had known. They always knew at least two weeks or more prior to the auditor's arrival. They had had this privilege for years. I learned there was some "inside information trading" going on. An employee of the Medical Records department would act as informant, warning our manager about "surprise" audits planned for UWP. I forgot that our manager had previously worked in medical records herself. She had connections. Stephen explained this had been the process for years. As soon as the medical records employee received the request from state auditors concerning specific medical files, reports needed, and planned weeks for their inspection, she would relay this information to Janine. UWP would always remain at least one step ahead of the auditors.

Stephen commented on the size of my chart load as I successfully navigated the cart in to our office. He immediately offered to assist with the unloading process. Megan volunteered as well. As we removed the last few charts, Janine entered our work quarters, seemingly unimpressed with the volume of charts I had.

"This is a lot of work people," Janine said. The charts were divided equally and we were reminded to look carefully for required reports. Janine handed each of us a photocopied list of needed information we were responsible for. Files with documentation issues were to be placed on a walnut colored desk in a designated corner. Janine would give those charts personal attention. Turning, she vanished from the room as if it had all been a dream.

Stephen snarled, wondering, "If that woman ever said thank you." I, too, had wondered that on many occasions.

"Go ask her," I teased. Megan looked on without saying a word. She appeared tired.

With the teasing aside, we knew it was time to turn serious. There was too much work to process and limited time to do it.

We lunged full speed into the charts, working almost in silence, each seemingly concerned the distraction of conversation would cause us to overlook needed reports. Two hours passed before I glanced at the wall clock again, and when I did I realized my shift would soon be over. Relieved, I glanced around and felt a sharp pain in my neck. Its tightness made me stop and inhale. "Ouch!"

Megan looked startled, immediately asking what had happened. Hearing a voice seemed strange at that moment. I explained that the stiffness in my neck was uncomfortable. It had been in a bended position too long.

For Megan, growing up with an uncle as a chiropractor had offered many advantages. One was learning terrific methods for massaging necks.

"Let me show you," she continued. I welcomed the offer.

Stephen teased that he wanted to be her next patient. Pretending to growl, Megan's hands went to work with the expertise of a pro. Closing my eyes, I began to relax, allowing Megan to massage away my tension. Relief was coming for the first time that day. However, that relief was short lived when I heard Janine's shrill tone demanding to know what was going on. There she stood, comparing what she was witnessing to a massage parlor. Seemingly embarrassed, Megan immediately began to explain.

"Swannee had pain in her neck. I was just trying to help," Megan explained. Janine was unconcerned and allowed the sarcasm in her tone to show.

Detecting the perfect time to change the subject, Stephen jumped in to the conversation, raving that we had processed all the files except for a few. Janine had a lot of work ahead of her because many of the files were missing adequate documentation.

Glancing around, Janine asked where the problem files were.

"On the back desk like you told us." Stephen said and pointed to the stack. Janine appeared confused, as if she had forgotten our previous conversation. She began to ramble that these charts were problems caused by the physicians and their inability to document when they were supposed to. She continued on, adding how much simpler our jobs would be if they would only do this. Appearing tired of hearing Janine's repetitive statements of complaint, Stephen pushed the conversation onward.

He agreed with her, but since this wasn't the case, something else needed to be done. There was a stack of charts she could begin working on. Realizing the mounting task, Janine offered a last minute change of plans. We were each instructed to divide the stacks equally and mail documentation requests to the various physicians. We were to see if we could get physicians to document the needed reports, or see if their secretaries would obtain the needed information and mail it to us. Our schedule was tight and we could only allow a week to acquire documentation. Reports needed to be found and placed in the designated area of the medical file. Everything must be exact. The urgency was heard in Janine's tone, and her eyes stressed the importance of this task as well. Dividing the charts, we began working on our new assignment. I finished filling out my last request form with ten minutes to spare in my work schedule. The day had been exhausting, and as I said my goodbyes, I wondered what the remainder of the week had in store for us. I assumed more of the same pressure.

The next week was filled with more tension-filled responsibilities. Glancing at my own work responsibilities that were piling up, I pondered if I would ever catch up. Luckily, the distraction of the audit kept Janine and upper management from calling too often about other delayed billing requests. At the end of the week Megan, Stephen and I compared notes on the reports we still needed to acquire. We had managed to obtain most of the ones we needed, but several failed to contain the necessary physician signature and we were running out of time. There were only a few days left before the auditors arrived, and we had no choice but to bring the files to Janine's attention.

Stephen left early for an appointment. He offered to go with us to talk to Janine the next day about problem charts and our current work status if we wanted to wait. His offer was tempting. Megan and I hesitated momentarily. It was as if we could read each other's minds because her voice spoke my exact thoughts.

"If Janine finds out we had these problems and could have given her an extra day to resolve them and didn't, she won't like it." I knew she was right.

This was not the time to hold back. I thought we should get things moving and reluctantly volunteered to go tell Janine. I sensed Megan's discomfort and didn't want to burden her. There was no one else to do it and other co-workers were dealing with other billing problems. It was time.

Stephen pretended to push me out the office door towards Janine's office, but I found little humor in this gesture. Giving him a final wave of the hand, I took a deep breath and walked across the hall. Twisting the knob, I tried my best to gather last minute ideas, but my mind felt blank.

Peering in to Janine's office I could see that she and Monica were engrossed in conversation as they sipped their daily cups of coffee. Their cackling annoyed me. Why should their day appear so relaxing when the rest of us were stressed to the max? The click of the door caused a synchronized head turn. I tried to smile and apologized profusely for interrupting their conversation. Janine appeared to disregard the disruption until the mention of audit charts caused a serious look to grace her face.

Motioning with her hand, it became evident that it was time for Monica to leave. Monica's look of irritation amused me as she gathered her belongings. Following her, Janine and I trekked the short walk towards my office. Megan was waiting beside the pile of charts. She stood, poised and speechless, awaiting Janine's review of the chart pile. What to do next? Who knew? All we could do was wait. It soon became obvious Janine was worried, as she commented on the size of the stack.

Did she think this was news to us? I thought silently. I felt frustrated because we seemed to be the ones doing all the work.

I explained our status. Requests had been sent to physicians for documentation, but we had not received any responses. Since it was nearing the time for the auditors to come, "we thought it best to inform you," Megan added.

Janine felt we had done the right thing by informing her. Flipping through a few of the top charts, she seemed distracted momentarily. Biting her lower lip, Janine asked me for the daily patient log. I advised her that it was across the hall with Darcy. Turning immediately, she headed in that direction.

Megan and I glanced back and forth at each other, confused. How a sheet showing what patients had been admitted into the hospital the previous night and to what department would help her was beyond comprehension at the moment. She didn't seem too concerned about our thoughts. Within minutes she returned with the list in hand. Sitting at Stephen's desk, she grabbed the telephone and began frantically pounding the keys. She was calling Medical Records and we listened closely as she began to speak.

"Thank you," she said before slamming the receiver down. Medical Records had pulled all their requested files for the day, but they were willing to do another special pull for us. Megan and I nodded, pretending to understand where this conversation was heading. I was given a list with fifteen patient names on them and instructed to get as many of the files as possible. Once collected, they were to be given to Janine. An hour later, a telephone call from Medical Records informed us our files were ready for pickup. Megan dashed up to get them, much to my relief, as Janine came to our office and sat down at Stephen's empty desk once again. Rushing in with the new stack of charts shortly thereafter, Megan's face appeared flushed. Her quickened breathing indicated she had rushed—every minute counted. Taking the pile we had previously made and combining those files with the new ones, Janine began rapidly searching the charts. Opening Stephen's side desk drawer, she rummaged through it, searching for something. Pulling out a pair of scissors and scotch tape, Janine began cutting, flipping, and taping. What was happening remained unclear, but at least Megan and I were free to finish some of our own job responsibilities.

*Scrunch, scrunch, scrunch...*the scissors cut through pieces of paper again and again. The sound of tape ripping filled the air, and as Janine applied tape to a sheet of paper, she hummed aloud, baffling me. Going to the photocopier, she raised the lid, slid in a piece of paper and pressed start. The printed page was heard dropping into the side tray. Grabbing it, she stared. Suddenly her face lit up like a beacon beckoning a lost ship in the fog.

"Perfect!" she said. "Absolutely perfect!" Looking around the room, she glanced at us motioning, for us to come take a look. Standing beside her, I looked in astonishment. I could feel Megan's glare penetrating the side of my face. Our limbs were frozen. There before us was a perfectly produced copy of a documented report, complete with *all* the necessary physician signatures. Our minds were racing, attempting to determine how it had all transformed. Momentarily, her guilt captivated her, compelling her to explain her actions.

She began speaking slowly, as if attempting to gain sympathy. Janine used the current patient roster to gather patient names and account numbers from particular medical departments. Comparing names to the stack of problem charts, she took a patient from the list that had been previously admitted to the same department, assuming she would find the needed physician signature somewhere in the chart.

"Guess what?" she asked as if we were playing a game. Neither one of us responded, so she continued on. A report the doctor had previously signed was carefully photocopied. The signature was then cut out neatly in a square and taped onto the report that it was needed on. *Voila!* The doctor had miraculously signed the report, and we instantaneously had the necessary documentation needed. Unsure of the proper response with this stunning revelation, Megan and I stood there, dumbfounded. Returning to our seats, we returned to work in a "zombie-like" state; there was nothing left to say.

Except for an occasional profee coordinator popping into the office to check their mailbox, almost thirty minutes passed in utter silence. Their smiles heightened my stress level. They hadn't seen what had occurred; therefore, their unawareness prevented them from experiencing my emotions.

Monica entered the room to check her mailbox and asked how things were going. It was clear her question was geared towards Janine. Neither Megan nor I bothered to respond.

Janine's "terrific" response was enthusiastic. Monica's facial expression revealed surprise. It wasn't long ago her friend had appeared worried. Obviously something had changed. Monica seemed joyful that her friend was feeling better. Tossing the last traces of her evident deception into a nearby garbage can, Janine left her stack of completed charts on the edge of Stephen's desk. She and Monica were taking a coffee break and she informed us that the pile would be completed upon her return. Her menacing stare seemed to have a hidden meaning meant for two: Megan and I. The two of them left the room, engaged in a conversation about a new recipe they wanted to try.

Stephen greeted me with a cheerful "good morning" the following day. I could tell from his reaction that Megan had failed to share what we had witnessed the previous evening. I didn't blame her, and I was unsure if I would say anything myself. Janine's unvoiced threat lingered in my mind. The thought of facing her wrath gave me chills. However, Stephen sensed something was out of sync and continued to ask questions until we reluctantly shared what we had witnessed. His eyes inflated at the stunning revelation as he questioned the seriousness of the information just shared. This was no joke, he soon learned, and we immediately warned him that the information must stay between the three of us.

Trying to convince us that someone must be told about this situation, my anger began to boil. He had known about the audit transactions, but hadn't reported it. His comment sounded hypocritical.

Controlling my emotions, I explained, "It is our word against hers. You know how management sticks together."

He nodded his understanding and discussed the seriousness of this scenario. Megan sat in silence, listening to the conversation, but her eyes looked fearful. What could we do? Just then Janine entered the room, bringing our brief conversation to an immediate halt. Her gaze was questioning, but gave away nothing. She inquired if everything was ok, to which we immediately replied "yes" in unison. Did she believe we would tell her if it weren't?

"That's what I want to hear," Janine shot back. Her conversation then turned towards the stress the audit had brought into her life. It had the same affect on all of us, but that appeared to be of little concern to her. Stephen glanced in my direction, but I ignored his gaze. Unsure of what to do, I didn't want to stir up trouble, and from Megan's reaction I could tell she was in agreement.

We were reminded that the auditors would arrive the next day and we were warned to be on our best behavior. If they had questions, it was our responsibility to ensure they had everything they needed. Our head movement indicated that we understood the instructions clearly.

Ms. Charlene Robinson was led into our office. Janine explained that Charlene was conducting our Medicare audit. Following Janine closely, this stout, thirty-something-looking female appeared serious as she firmly gripped a small leather business bag. Her expression chilled me and I wondered what the atmosphere would be like as she worked. She was guided towards a small work area behind my desk. I attended classes in the morning, so while I was at school she would use my desk to conduct her business.

With the formalities complete, Janine instructed me to assist where needed, and if there were problems to bring them to her attention. I had heard those statements consistently lately; they were beginning to sound rehearsed.

I responded with a rehearsed "absolutely" comment, managing somehow to plaster a smile across my face. Ms. Robinson sat down and immediately began working. She made small talk, but appeared focused.

I issued a final reminder for her to ask if there was anything she needed.

"Thank you," she replied. Her face suddenly looked gentle under the glare of the desk lamp. For an hour she worked in silence and the disruption of her soft-spoken voice made me jump with a start. I had forgotten she was behind me.

Apologizing for startling me, her hand came to a resting place upon my shoulder as if to comfort me. Attempting to regain my composure, I smiled.

The truth was I had been jumpy for the past couple of days. Ms. Robinson was searching for a cytology report she had been unable to locate.

Relaxing, that was a question I could easily answer.

"Those are behind the pathology tab in the file. The reports have a pink border." Flipping through the file, I instantly found the one she was searching for. Glancing at the report, I recognized it as one containing our trademark method of documentation practice. Throughout the years I had noticed that often the pathology reports failed to contain the name of the pathologist indicated on claim forms (HCFA) we processed our work from. From the beginning of my UWP employment, I had been trained to type the physicians name on the report because "that is the way it has always been done." I wondered now if that was legally acceptable, but I didn't know. I wasn't about to direct this question to the auditor. I still knew what I had witnessed earlier couldn't ever be legal. Pointing out a few last details, Charlene easily grasped the concepts I explained and seemed genuinely appreciative.

I relaxed and the two of us chatted for several minutes, managing to share an occasional laugh. Janine and Monica entered the room as we talked freely and her eyes darted from face to face, searching for an answer to the question, *what is going on here?* Feeling uncomfortable at having been caught during a light-hearted moment, I reapplied my business face. Charlene detected the change and voluntarily explained to Janine and Monica how helpful I had been and how appreciative she was. Janine looked relieved and smiled like a proud parent. The remainder of Charlene's days auditing our department went well. As I suspected, the *chart documentation was outstanding*.

Saying goodbye to Charlene on her final day at the office was almost unbearable; Megan, Stephen, and I stood at full attention smiling. My plastered smile weighed heavily upon my conscience. I needed to talk to someone about what was happening within the department—someone who had the power to eliminate this witnessed deception. I needed to tell John.

That afternoon as Janine and Laurie Brooks—another hospital worker—departed for an in-house meeting, I knew this provided ample time for me to make my call. Waiting for my call to transfer, I realized I had intentionally disguised my voice when asking for John. I didn't want anyone to know I was calling John and cause problems. Lately the company grapevine had been working overtime.

John wasn't available. The voice on the other end of the receiver was unrecognizable and I didn't dare ask for their name, frightened they might do the same.

I refused to leave a message. That was too great a risk.

"No thank you," I whispered into the receiver. I hadn't told Megan and Stephen I was calling John and was unsure yet if I would. I tried to reach John again within an hour.

After the click of the telephone was heard, I held the receiver momentarily, unsure what to do next.

Megan observed me holding the telephone sans conversation and asked if I was okay.

"Everything is just fine," I replied, sounding enthusiastic. The conversation changed to the audit and the relief we felt that it was over. *Yeah, but was it really?* I wondered. An hour later I telephoned John again, only to find he remained unavailable. Now I had no choice but to wait. Janine would be returning soon. I wouldn't attempt a third call. Of all days, why did he have to pick today to be so *unavailable?* Something had to change, and soon.

Half an hour later the telephone rang, and I reached for it instantly. It wouldn't be John calling; he didn't know I was looking for him, but I silently prayed he might be calling Janine. Instead, I was surprised to hear my own mother's voice, sharing some disappointing news. Her current employer was going to close within a week. Shocked, I hung up the telephone, wondering how I could help. My answer arrived a month later, with the posting of a full-time position. Reading the job description, I became wide-eyed. Turning to stare at Stephen, I inhaled. It was *his* job. What was going on?

Approaching Stephen for an explanation, he informed me the company had recently decided to add lead positions at the hospitals (University and Harborview) because management responsibilities were increasing. He applied, and was offered the position.

I pressed him for an explanation. This was the first I had heard about this. Megan's startled expression showed she had no idea about the current events either.

Stephen leaned back in his chair, frantically searching for an acceptable explanation. It was upsetting. We had all been close friends for so long, it remained unclear why he had failed to mention this. Silence engulfed the room for several seconds; Megan and I shrugged our shoulders as a peaceful gesture.

Looking in my direction, he began the process of convincing me that this would work out well for me as well. I failed to catch his meaning. He continued, explaining that the vacancy of his position approaching would leave a full-time job available for me.

The thought of applying for his job made me nervous and was unappealing. There was already too much stress and deception occurring within the company. Why would I want to work full time for UWP?

Stephen continued making his case by reminding me that I would be graduating from college before I realized it and searching for a full-time job. This statement was factual, and I hated to agree with him. He suggested adjusting my school schedule and grabbing this full-time job while it was available. Despite the validity of his argument, I was hesitant. I knew too many of the inexcusable business operations, but in the back of my mind I could hear my mothers voice saying "I will be out of work soon." I needed to take this job. We needed the money.

Unable to resist the temptation, Megan asked what my decision was. She appeared hopeful that I would go for it. It would also ensure she had a true friend to talk to confidentially about what was going on.

Taking a deep breath, I said, "I'm going to apply for the job." They both smiled, happy with my decision. I was unsure I was.

Within a month Janine called me to her office for a different reason. Smiling, Janine offered me a full-time position with UWP. This conversation didn't seem real, but I accepted her offer. Placing a manila envelope in my hand, Janine presented a sincere sounding "Congratulations! You have just become a full time UWP employee." I smiled back at her. An inner-office celebration occurred the following morning in my honor. Fruit, donuts, bagels, and the aroma of fresh coffee filled the room. Congratulatory welcomes, one after the other, greeted me from co-workers.

"You're one of us," they chanted. At that moment, looking around at the many wonderful faces I had grown to know through the years, I truly felt proud.

Professional Fee Coordinator: Mark Erickson

A change happened within our department with the hiring of Professional Fee Coordinator Mark Erickson. This attractive mixture of Caucasian, Filipino, Norwegian male was an almost immediate distraction to several department females. His initial shyness seemed to prevent him from noticing the affect he had on the opposite sex. Most of his breaks and lunchtime were spent with a female co-worker, Darcy, who was intent on establishing a close relationship. After joining them one afternoon for lunch, I began to notice that his mood was relaxing. I found his personality comical and as the three of us talked for an hour, I discovered that Mark and I had a lot in common and felt we would form a friendship as well.

It wasn't long before Mark began to notice the same documentation problems I had when I had first started working for the company. Approaching me, he pressed me on how these situations were handled within the organization. Relaying as much information to him as I could about the billing practices and resolutions, I was careful to make sure management didn't overhear us. Documentation and billing problems were well known throughout the University based employees of UWP, but it was still a taboo subject for discussion. Raising too many issues about problems could acquire you unwelcome attention from Janine. She knew she held the power within the group and seized every opportunity to remind you.

One Friday afternoon, Mark questioned me about the method for handling missing documentation after flipping through a chart repeatedly, in search of patient progress notes. His frustration mounted by the minute as he reminded me that the attending physician was supposed to document a patient's chart every three days. That's how they told the patient's current health status. Mark complained of already having too much work. It was ridiculous to think he could go around chasing after information for each patient. "There is no way doctors could have gotten away with this at my old employer," he practically shouted.

I reminded him that he had entered a new world of billing with their set of rules. There was the right way, and then there was the University Physicians way of doing things. He would learn the routine soon enough. I informed him I had been asking everyone around here about policies for years. No one wanted to hear it. I felt there was nothing we could do about it. His look seemed to shoot daggers at me. I apologized, sympathetic to his frustration. I had reached that point long ago. It was very frustrating for the abstractors, too. Motioning for him to follow me, we headed around the corner to briefly continue our conversation.

Profee coordinators were instructed to bill for surgical procedures by using progress notes. This made it very difficult for abstractors to do their jobs. "If an insurance company is looking for an operative report and it isn't in the chart, who do you think has to go find it and put it in the chart?" I questioned. Mark looked puzzled, and from that day on I knew I had found another avenue to voice my concern about business practices within the department.

Mark asked about my friendship with John Reed, believing that might be a successful outlet for making changes. Explaining that we had some mutual friends, his face appeared disheartened when I explained this route had previously been attempted unsuccessfully.

"He doesn't seem very interested in hearing about it. John has so many other responsibilities that he doesn't want to deal with something like this—something that seems so minor," I explained. Mark argued that this wasn't minor; it was a problem. I understood all too well. With John having so many people to answer to, I believed he viewed these issues as things we could handle.

My other concern, I confessed to Mark, was that I didn't want him to think I was ungrateful. He did tell me about this job and I was smart enough to realize I made very good money for someone my age. Raising an eyebrow, Mark responded with a smirk and teased me about hearing a rumor when he first started that I was "given" my job. Defensive, I explained I might have received help getting my foot in the door, but I was the one handling the work responsibilities I had been assigned to. I couldn't help but allow the frustration of his comment to show. I was hurt. He knew I knew my job, and the look of sorrow upon his face showed he wished he had remained silent for that portion of the conversation.

With work demands and responsibilities on the rise, I made myself a promise to talk privately with John when I had an opportunity. I needed to be straightforward and lay everything on the line once and for all. We knew each other well enough to talk comfortably. I would ask him to hold our conversation in confidence. The following Wednesday he was scheduled to attend a meeting with the Dean for the UW School of Medicine. Sans Janine in the office, I knew it would be easy to pull him aside for a private discussion. John was predictable; he would stop by to see how things were going prior to the meeting. I could approach him then, but things didn't work out as planned. The phone rang shortly after noon with a fast-paced telephone call from John's secretary. He had felt ill earlier that morning, gone to the emergency room, and been diagnosed as having had a heart attack. Janine returned to the department a few hours later with an update. John would be on medical leave for the next month. I would remain silent about any concerns I had. I had to. There was no one else in upper management I felt comfortable enough talking to. I still enjoyed my job, but things on the inside were beginning to change too rapidly for me.

The following morning, a staff meeting was called and we were briefed on our billing expectations. Since John was Janine's boss, she emphasized the importance of prioritizing our job responsibilities and remaining productive, as always. He didn't need the stress, she reiterated. Staff members detected her message as a threat. I pitied the individual who dared to mess up.

Work processing continued as usual, but in a move that stunned the entire staff Darcy was promoted from abstractor to professional fee coordinator. This move made no sense. The Medicaid position proved challenging for her, and to advance to major billing responsibilities was practically a death sentence for Janine. What was she thinking? Allowing her to bill for one of the most difficult, confusing, services in the hospital: Neurosurgery. Many of the hospital's neurosurgeons had reputations that preceded them. Their sternness and continual demands for answers on billing practices from Janine made them a department no one wanted to deal with. A large percentage of the staff feared these physicians. Others claimed they had a "God complex." To have the talent and ability to perform such complex surgical procedures daily, I assumed they would almost have to. I admired them. When it came to University Physician management, these doctors had no fear.

Darcy stepped into her new position with a huge smile and several speeches about her determination to succeed. Everyone knew she was in over her head, and that included Janine most of all. Many wondered why she had chosen Darcy. I soon discovered the answer. During one of our casual conversations in the office, Janine shared information with us about her upcoming planned European vacation, scheduled to start the following week. Her excitement was felt throughout the room. We were all happy she would be gone, too, because that meant a more relaxed work environment for us. Stephen had become a carefree department head. With him in charge of our department during Janine's absence, it would be just like managing ourselves. In a sense, we would all get a vacation; some of us just wouldn't have to leave town to do so.

One afternoon, as Janine stood using our office photocopier, she asked how I had learned to do my job so well. I was surprised by her question and taken aback by the compliment she had managed to slip in. Through the years, employees had learned that most major work compliments were given during your annual employee evaluation.

"Thank you. I had a lot of on-the-job training and wonderful support here. I didn't really know anything about this field when I started, but the more hands-on experience you get, the easier it becomes. I took plenty of notes, used a repetition technique, and reviewed everything I learned. Now it is like second nature. I am comfortable," I explained.

She was straightforward about her recognition of people's surprise at the selection of Darcy for the Neurosurgery profee coordinator position. I remained expressionless.

What Janine shared next stunned me and will stay with me forever. She explained that Darcy wasn't the best candidate, but she wanted the position. There was no one else interested in the job. Because of the volume of surgical procedures occurring within that medical division, it wasn't wise to leave it vacant for any length of time. The position needed to be filled.

I nodded to indicate I was listening. She continued on. "If you can learn all you did, I know she can too," Janine stated, sounding convincing. I smiled, wondering if that statement was made for my benefit or hers.

Our eyes met as I digested all she had just said. I knew Darcy was a wonderful, intelligent person, but it was unfair to put her in the position of being compared to someone else. We were different individuals. Our work ethics were different. Who would take the blame if she wasn't successful in her new position? A part of me didn't want to know the answer to that question.

Tracey entered the office with irritability visible upon her face. Holding a chart, she tossed it onto the medical cart, grabbed a paper cup and went to the water jug. For several minutes she remained there, quietly accepting the welcome coolness the water brought. Turning to face me, she began to reveal a problem I had heard too much.

She was attempting to bill for a surgical procedure. It was a co-surgery. This meant she couldn't process her portion of the bill until the neurosurgery charges had been coded and billed. Her cheeks were rosy. I was well aware this had happened as she attempted to regain her composure. Tracey had been a professional fee coordinator for three years and she prided herself in staying on top of her work responsibilities. She was familiar with billing for several departmental services and was particularly well respected by the Orthopedic Department. Her rapport with the orthopedic physicians was terrific because it was important for the physicians to have their charges processed in a timely manner. The more charges submitted to the various insurance companies, the larger the reimbursement. In addition, the larger the dollar amount that was billed for a department, the larger the additional monies received. Hospital physicians received a percentage of whatever dollar amounts their departments billed. Money was everything.

It was the dollar amounts that were causing a problem for Tracey today. It was the ongoing battle with Darcy that had commenced almost from the moment she had become a profee coordinator. It was common knowledge within the department—Tracey was one of the fastest billing coordinators. Any deadlines she was required to meet were always met and quality work was presented. If you required assistance, she was available. She managed issues with any of the physicians she billed for comfortably, discussed problems openly, and stood her ground when necessary until an agreeable solution was reached. Staff members admired her, many wishing they could be as forthcoming. However, from the beginning Janine found her to be trouble, and the two often clashed.

Twelve years separated us in age, but we became fast friends. In many ways Tracey became my mentor. If I knew an issue needed to be presented to the staff, I could tell her about it; she would present it without indicating I was the one who had the concern. She had reached a work-and-growth level that I aspired to reach. On this day, I watched as I had so many times before; she took the last few gulps of her water and headed across the hall towards Janine's office. I knew a battle was about to unfold.

It wasn't long before Mark scurried over to our office with his familiar smirk on his face. This was a clear indication something major was happening.

"What?" I asked. The urgency in my voice was evident. I didn't give him much eye contact. Through the years we had all learned it was best to appear busy, even if you weren't. Removing several pages from a folder he held in his hand, I gave him my attention briefly. My ears awaited the details of what he had witnessed.

"All hell broke loose," he commenced.

A slight gasp escaped my lips. Tracey always stood her ground for what she believed in. Janine would never succeed in intimidating her, no matter how hard she tried. There was a part of me that envied that. Tracey worked her job by choice. The mother of three sons, her husband made enough money to support her in the event she decided to quit her job. Most staff members worked their jobs because they had to. Janine was aware of this and often reminded personnel "anyone off the street can come in and do this job." That wasn't true. To perform our jobs required plenty of training. We prided ourselves in our skills, abilities and the standards we upheld, but hearing this belittlement repeatedly affected the self-esteem of many and created an environment of workers lacking enthusiasm.

Tracey had been summoned to Janine's office for a meeting. Janine had recently learned that Tracey had held a meeting with one of her departmental physicians without informing her. She was furious. Janine needed to know *everything* that happened in the department.

I couldn't understand why Tracey meeting with one of her departmental physicians would anger Janine. I would think she would want her to stay on top of any billing issues. What I failed to see was that Janine felt threatened by anyone making decisions without her input. Janine needed to be in control of the department. Within minutes Tracey made her way back into our office. Everything about her face showed the anger she felt. The beet color in her complexion gave the impression of someone about to lose control. No one spoke for several seconds. Tracey finally broke the silence.

The environment was beginning to take its toll on Tracey. I had never witnessed her allowing a situation to control her like this, and for the first time she informed us she didn't know how much longer she would be staying with the company. She detailed her feelings of frustrations about giving her all on a daily basis, but nothing was ever good enough. We were all still forced to face a tremendous amount of criticism. Luckily for Tracey, she had a few options:

stay, find a new job, or become a stay-at-home mother. I didn't want to know what her choice would be just yet.

Her words were frightening. I had never seen her this angry. I panicked. "We need you here," I said, interrupting her speech before she could continue her tirade. Through the months I had worked for the company, Tracey's determination and support was what had encouraged several of us. We depended on her for so many things; I don't think she ever realized how much.

Six months later I had the opportunity to tell Tracey how much she meant to us. After a brief meeting with Janine and a physician whose billing she handled, she had heard enough insults and said she no longer desired to be a part of UWP. I returned from a restroom trip to a *shock*. Tracey had turned in her resignation five minutes beforehand. Two weeks left on her commitments to the company and she was gone. We were terrified. What now?

Packing her belongings, Tracey said her goodbyes to staff members she had befriended through the years. Her face appeared joyous. Having recently added new financial responsibilities in my personal life, I looked on, knowing I needed to maintain my employment with UWP, but how the rest of us in room C214 would be treated after her departure worried me. I sat in silence, wondering.

A Startling Discovery

With Tracey gone, things settled down nicely. Janine was joyous, and for the first time in a while her mood was relaxed. Janine attended weekly meetings and luncheons at the main office. How we looked forward to those days, knowing from past experience it would be an all day event. Feedback on how the department was progressing, statistical information…it was all presented to upper management during those meetings. Several days prior to her meetings, Janine paced around the office, ensuring that she was prepared as she reviewed responses to potential questions. Her primary goal during those meetings was to create a flawless appearance for her staff members.

Popping her head inside the entrance of our office door, Janine informed us she was leaving for a meeting. A quick wave and she was gone. The usual *rat ta ta, rat ta tat* playing its rhythm was heard as she descended down the hallway. This was one day we could have a casual lunch and a little relaxation ourselves. Glancing around the office, I could tell that everyone intended to do just that.

My intercom buzzed, slightly startling me. Looking down, I recognized Mark's number. The tone of his voice indicated something was going on. He had something to show me and I told him I would be there momentarily. The urgency in his voice aroused my curiosity. I had five minutes remaining of my break, but I surmised that if I went over a little it wouldn't matter. Putting my purse into my desk drawer, I informed Stephen, who was sorting papers, that I would be across the hall if needed. He could be heard counting, but his nod indicated he had heard me.

Opening the door to the office across the hall, Mark motioned for me to hurry.

"What's the rush?" I asked, wondering what all the secrecy was about. He was the only one working in the room at the time and Janine wasn't expected to return until later that day.

Handing me a log sheet, his finger pointed at a certain spot. I scrolled down the page, looking at charges being billed for kidney dialysis treatment on a patient. Mark had circled one line on the page. I was puzzled. Handing me his calendar, he tapped with his index finger, motioning for me to look closer. I did. Mark had written a note. Everything became clear. Something was terribly wrong. There was no way the physician could bill for the services he had listed. During that time period, he *was out of the country.*

My mouth flew open and our eyes met, each apparently stunned. Placing my hand on his shoulder I asked, "How is this possible? This is something you have to bring to Janine's attention. This cannot be done." I knew his calendar dates were accurate, because it was common knowledge many hospital physicians willingly provided their profee coordinators with dates they would be on vacation.

Mark decided to discuss this startling discovery with Janine upon her return. Shrugging his shoulders, I noticed his right eyebrow was elevated. I had known him long enough to know this indicated something was up. I, too, had my suspicions.

Stephen walked in, allowing his sarcasm to come as well. He had recently coined the term "lovebirds" when referring to us. I found this particularly offensive, since everyone else understood our friendship. Eyeing us suspiciously, he walked towards Janine's room and tossed a chart on her desk. Mark and I glanced at him, feeling slightly irritated by his intrusion and comment. His mannerisms had changed over the past weeks following his promotion. He seemed pleased to view himself as a senior employee, and the fun, gentle guy I once enjoyed working with so much had become an annoyance to many.

"We were just finishing, thank you," I chimed. I slid the paper back towards Mark to put away before Stephen could approach his desk. Opening the door, I left the room without saying another word or glancing back. Minutes later, Stephen returned to our office, seemingly content at having ended any discussion Mark and I were involved in. I didn't care. My thoughts raced elsewhere. I wanted to know what Janine would say about the billing. Would she actually allow a doctor to charge without being present? I would have to wait for my answer.

A ringing telephone, sounds of paper shuffling, and the rattle of the copier indicated our work environment was once again in full swing. I struggled to remain focused on my job responsibilities. A nagging sensation continued to distract me. I refused to discuss this new concern with other staff members because it seemed useless. I had been working in the organization long enough to know where the true power of the company lay: hospital physicians, upper management, and middle management. Stephen glanced in my direction several times, noticing that something was distracting me. Avoiding his gaze, I remained silent with my thoughts of worry.

The sound of Janine's return caught my attention instantaneously. Now was the moment of truth. I heard the click of her office door as it closed behind her. Mark must be talking to her and I expected to hear my intercom buzzing shortly. I knew Mark ran the risk of having his conversation overheard if he attempted to telephone me. I, too, ran that same risk. Plenty of time had passed. Mark must know something by now. My patience was running out. Just then the shrill sound of the intercom jolted me! Answering quickly, I expected to hear Marks' voice, but I was surprised to hear Janine's instead.

Her voice sounded cold and emotionless as she spoke, requesting that I come to her office. Hanging up the phone, I was nervous. I was sure she knew Mark and I had been discussing billing problems. Somehow Stephen must have told her. She must be irritated, and probably had already taken her frustrations out on Mark. Now it was my turn. Approaching the door, I ran a few excuses through my mind.

"Sorry, Janine, I was just trying to..." No I couldn't start with the word sorry, that would indicate I had done something wrong. Try again. "Mark asked me to look at..." No, no that wasn't the correct start either. I would just go with her lead and take it from there. I had done nothing wrong. Taking one last deep breath, I turned the doorknob and entered. Glancing at Mark, sitting at his desk, I tried to read his eyes, but they were focused on a medical file.

Janine motioned me into her office with her right index finger. I entered and was relieved when she asked me to deliver a chart to Medical Records for her. This tradition had started with the departure of Louise. Chart delivery to other departments was a "petty task that could be handled by the abstractors." I had overheard Louise explaining this to Janine when she became manager. I found the comment insulting. However, this time it was a welcome relief and I eagerly accepted the chart. Considering an alternative conversation was chilling. Leaving the room for the second time, I attempted to make eye contact with Mark, but he avoided my gaze. His message was unclear, but I knew I could take other measures to find out what was going on.

Making my way towards Marcella's office, I knocked, preparing to ask if I could use the telephone. Marcella had been a hospital employee for over ten years and occupied an office on the third floor. There was no response, but I knew it was okay to enter. She had always told me I was welcome to use her telephone anytime I needed privacy. She knew it was difficult to have any privacy in our office. Closing the door behind me, I picked up the telephone and dialed the extension to my office. Clearing my throat, I heard Stephen's voice offer a greeting. Attempting to sound professional and stifling a laugh, I pulled out my best southern accent and asked for Mark.

Stephen wanted to know who was calling. *He's so damn nosy*, I thought, *always wanting to know Mark's business.*

"It's Veronica." I giggled. Confusion was evident in Mark's voice as he answered the phone. I was sure he was attempting to figure out who Veronica was.

I wasted no time in letting him know Veronica's true identity. He chuckled slightly. His tone then turned serious. That let me know he wasn't alone. He knew what information I was searching for.

"Did you get a chance to ask Janine about the billing scenario?" I pressed on.

Pretending to discuss a medical issue, I awaited details.

"And?" I continued, wanting him to hurry.

It was then that I learned he had been instructed to proceed with his billing.

"*What?*" I shouted into the stillness of the room.

Repeating the information once more, I remained on the telephone, speechless. There was nothing more to say. I could do nothing except clutch the receiver. Exiting Marcella's office, I made my way through the busy hospital corridor, feeling sad. The company I had once loved so much was changing even more than I realized.

Deceptive Billing Practices

Our departmental staff meeting came to order. Janine flipped through a few pages in her notebook. All was quiet except for the creaking of a chair. Though not held consistently, whenever management felt there was something worth discussing we would gather for this spur-of-the-moment event. Today, topics to be covered were coding issues, inconsistencies with billing policies amongst the staff, and upper management concerns that were presented. *Boring* was all I could think. These meetings rarely included anything for the abstractors and I felt our time could be better spent processing paperwork. Still, we were all required to attend. I sat there, listening to see if anything would grasp my attention. This time something did. A new policy was being implemented about handling the billing for operative procedures. Previously, billing was not to occur if sufficient documentation wasn't available and in the medical file. But, effective immediately, if the patient was on the hospital log as being admitted to have a procedure, the professional fee coordinator was to proceed with the billing and process paperwork whether documentation was available or not. If insurance companies needed documentation later, then an abstractor would handle the request. My job responsibilities had just changed to include that of a medical detective. Sitting there lifeless, the burden of this added responsibility became apparent upon the faces of the abstractors. The department currently housed only three abstractors, but what could we say?

Janine attempted to sound encouraging by reminding us that there was a strong possibility that particular reports wouldn't be requested by an insurance company or auditor. I knew too many wrong doings would merely lead to disaster.

Why were things proceeding this way? I wondered.

As the meeting progressed, I learned more complaints were coming from physicians regarding the timeliness of getting their charges billed. The larger a dollar amount that was billed by a department, the larger their additional monies or incentive checks would be. Attending physicians of the University Hospital received a base salary, and in addition a percentage of what their department collected. This amount often escalated into additional thousands of dollars monthly. I had never viewed the dollar amount on a check, but this fact was known throughout the department. Incentive checks were delivered at the end of each month. Calls were received promptly from physicians during this time, requesting the status of their expectant checks. The urgency in their voices stressed the importance of receiving theses monies.

The following month incentive checks arrived, but the department was short-staffed and I was called to assist with the delivery to the various departments. After sorting the checks by their floors (room numbers), I noticed one piece of paper at the bottom of the delivery box. Looking to see what it was, I gasped. It was a physician check that somehow hadn't been placed in an envelope. Looking at it, I was *speechless at the dollar amount*. Worth slightly more than $10,000, this was the largest check value I recalled ever touching. Heading across the hall towards Janine's office, I knew I better give it to her. Reviewing it, I could tell she was impressed by its value as well.

I was instructed to place the check in a clean envelope and deliver it to the physician's office as usual. Trembling, I went from floor to floor, delivering envelopes. I now realized why physicians wanted those checks so desperately. While photocopying notes from a chart later that afternoon, Janine came in and teased me about the dollar amount on the check we had seen earlier. We were both in agreement that it would be nice to know a check that size was coming for you at the end of each month.

John popped his head into the room, greeting us with his usual smile. He wanted to know how everything was going. I now knew the truth; he just wanted to hear there were no problems.

"Good," I commented. What else was I to say?

Janine had papers for him and briskly headed towards her office to retrieve them.

Sitting in an empty chair beside my desk, John started making small talk.

"How's your mother?" he questioned.

"Very well, thank you."

I was truly happy to see that John had returned to work and was feeling better, and I told him so. The doctors expected him to make a full recovery as long as he didn't overdo anything. Smiling sheepishly, I decided to take a chance and told John I had tried to reach him several times before he got sick. I wanted to talk to him privately when he had time. He looked puzzled and he offered to sit for a few minutes to chat. Frantically shaking my head no, it became obvious to John that this was not the place to do it.

Slipping me his home telephone number, I stressed we could talk about 7:00 p.m. that evening. Just then Janine reentered the room. She looked worried when she saw John sitting at my desk. Aware of our pre UWP friendship, she seemed consistently worried I would reveal too much information about the work environment. Reapplying my best professional face, I politely ended our conversation. There was no need to arouse suspicions. John was unfazed by her presence; he was the boss.

Taking the papers from Janine's hand, he politely thanked her and prepared to exit.

Giving a final glance over his shoulder, he bid us "goodbye" and was on his way.

Our sentiments echoed the same.

As John descended down the hallway, I turned my attention back to the stack of papers on my desk. Janine's eyes were riveted on me, but I ignored them. I was sure she wondered what we were discussing and as I tried to focus, I prayed she wouldn't ask.

Five, six, seven…the final digits of John's home number were dialed and as I waited for an answer I thought to myself that perhaps I shouldn't be making this call. What was I going to say? I would just make an excuse and call a different day, but it was too late. John's soft-spoken voice could be heard. Somehow I managed to respond and as I did, I detected a welcoming tone and curiosity in his voice. With small talk aside, we jumped right to the root of the problem. I informed John of several things that were going on within the department: treatment of employees, documentation issues, and invalid billings. His tone rang surprised, as if I had just said something totally absurd.

Informing me that this was the first he had heard about major documentation problems within our department, I concealed my disbelief. Explaining that Janine had been asked numerous times how things were going within the hospital, her response was "everything is under control." *I sat on the other end of the telephone, growing angrier by the minute.* The longer I talked to John, the more I realized that was all he wanted to hear. He was a nice man, but he didn't want any hassles in the work place. Politely ending our conversation, I asked him to keep this call between us. He assured me of his confidentiality. Replacing the telephone on the receiver, one thought raced through my mind: how could Janine say those words? From what I saw on a daily basis, things were beginning to spiral out of control.

During the following weeks I thought John might tell Janine we had spoken. I soon relaxed when I realized nothing had been said. Lately the office appeared to remain in a continual state of flux. Stephen was moved to an upper floor office because Janine felt as a lead he required additional privacy. I welcomed the news. Soon Megan and I acquired a new office mate.

Transaction Discrepancies

Barbara was a pleasant woman, appearing to be in her mid-fifties. Her wildly-styled curly hair gave the appearance of a woman out of control, but she was anything but. The pleasantness she added to the room was soothing and we formed a special friendship within a short time. Having suffered minor nerve damage before joining the department, there were noted occasions when flare-ups prevented her normal speed in completing her job responsibilities. Since this was a major part of our job responsibilities, Megan and I worked together to make sure Barbara met her deadlines. At times Janine didn't know who was processing some of the work. She didn't need to.

Processing work was about to become more difficult when we learned our group's financial counselor, Linda, was resigning her position. Rumblings spread amongst staff members who were worried about impending changes. Whenever someone departed or received a promotion, the department consistently went through a shuffling of work responsibilities. I knew things were about to become stressful, not just for my co-workers, and me but also for the unborn child I was now carrying.

Recently I had begun to feel a burning sensation in my stomach. I knew it was nerves. Perhaps on the outside my emotions weren't clearly visible, but my unborn child knew the truth. The baby could feel my pain, had to carry my burdens, and I knew it was unfair. I loved this baby growing within me so much and vowed to protect it at all costs. Embracing my stomach gently, I gave my expanding midsection a gentle squeeze. I knew this was going to be a difficult journey.

I was now the senior abstractor of the group and along with that came several disadvantages. Within two weeks I was thrust into tackling the tasks of patients with physician billing questions and insurance problems. Someone was needed to assist patients as they sought answers, and I received the vote. They streamlined me in briskly. Many were pleasant, but as the problems escalated, so did their impatience. Addressing their questions, I began to notice consistent problems. The physician listed on the itemized bill *wasn't a physician who had treated them* during their visit. I gave them explanations I had been provided with during my training. When a patient came for treatment at the hospital, they were often seen and treated by a resident physician. The attending physician then oversees what the resident has done and bills for the work, because residents could not bill. This was the way the process worked according to UWP, and this was how I had been instructed to explain it. Years passed before I learned that residents could not bill because they receive a salary. Billing guidelines stated attending physicians must be present at some time during a procedure to bill for it.

Patients were often unaware they would receive *two sets of bills* when they came to the hospital. These extra charges were frustrating for many. The hospital charged for the usage of the room, equipment…and the physicians billed for their actual services. Some patients argued this was a "rip-off," and through the years I watched many patients turned over to collection agencies because they couldn't pay the unexpected charges from both sides of the hospital.

The weeks passed and I interacted more with patients; many I got to know on a first name basis. I noticed what appeared to be duplicate charges for patients receiving kidney dialysis treatment. Patients brought in their hospital bills and their physicians bills and as the two were placed side by side, I found particular charges odd and noted they had the same ICD9 code and CPT code. *It did appear the physician bill was charging for something the hospital had previously charged for.* I wasn't certain about my observation, because I wasn't as familiar with billing policies as professional fee coordinators in this service area. I thought it was best to receive a second, perhaps even a third opinion.

Taking a patient name and account number, I telephoned the main office, asking for assistance from the Patient Relations department. Thankfully, the patient had departed the area so I could speak freely. I voiced my concern and learned that this *was* a duplicate billing and it was something that would be too difficult to fix because there were so many accounts handled this way. "Just leave it alone," the voice rang through the telephone.

"Leave it alone?" I chimed. "I need to know what they expected me to tell the patient." I was advised to "say nothing." The explanation continued. UWP wanted me to state the patients insurance company had been billed and we were awaiting payment. Patient Relations walked me through the screen so I could observe the fact that the charges had been billed. That was truthful, but in my heart I realized they were still lying, even if it was by omission. If the patient needed to make payment arrangements that could easily be arranged. I couldn't believe what I heard. As I placed the telephone on the receiver, I felt a familiar sensation in my stomach, something all too familiar. But this time it was different. I had someone else to think about. Rubbing my stomach, I worried how this stress was affecting my unborn child. I didn't like it. I somehow had to get away from this.

The fragile-looking gray-haired patient Mrs. Jenkins hobbled in with the assistance of her maple-colored walking cane. She lowered her body into the seat next to my desk and awaited answers about the charges on her itemized statement. Regaining my composure, I restated what had been explained to me—minus the hardcore truth—while plastering an artificial smile on my face. I prayed she couldn't detect anything unusual. Apparently nothing was noticed. Her friendliness remained the same, which made me feel worse.

Hearing a story that was all too familiar, the guilt consumed me. Her income was limited to social security, so payment arrangements had to be made. Biting my lower lip, I went into my desk drawer and removed a payment arrangement slip. Dialing Louise's office number, I relayed information received from Mrs. Jenkins and worked out the lowest payment possible for her to pay. Once details were completed, Mrs. Jenkins seemed comfortable with the dollar amount. I felt only guilt. Louise reminded me as long as we were receiving something from the patient, that was all that mattered.

I prided myself with the accounts I knew how to handle, and was thrilled when I found refunds owed to patients. However, I soon discovered "refund" didn't always mean the patient or insurance company got their money back. One Friday afternoon, while reviewing some forms a patient had dropped off, I became interested in account notes on the comment screen (screen 9) of our computer system. Taking a closer look, I realized the patient had paid on some charges and his insurance company had paid on the same charges several weeks later. This meant the patient had a refund coming: a few hundred dollars. This was wonderful news. I couldn't wait to share the news with the patient who was expected to stop by later that afternoon. I knew it was best to recheck my findings before sharing this information with the patient. My joy was brought to an immediate halt.

I was informed by one of our departmental representatives that the patient wasn't to be told about these findings. Perhaps I had misread the noted information. Determining that I didn't understand departmental computer abbreviations as well as I thought, I questioned further. My readings of these abbreviations were fine. What I learned that day was that I was unfamiliar with another company practice, which was occasionally put into place. If a patient account maintained a credit balance and it was obvious they were continually in for treatment, those funds were often held, rather than continuously rebilling the patient. Many of these patients were recognized for making slow payments and this method assisted in keeping their accounts more current. If an insurance company payment changed the status and made the account current, then the same rule applied—with one difference. These monies were shifted on the computer to cover a charge or make a partial payment on another. Many patients never realized they had a credit balance on their account.

Double payments from insurance companies didn't present any problems, either. Occasionally two insurance companies paid the full amount of a charge for a patient. The supplemental insurance should acquire the refund, but that rarely happened. Those funds were routinely kept, and by simply moving the money, applying it to another charge or holding it for an expectant future charge and making a notation on our company comment screen, the discrepancy in the transaction was concealed.

Why not give the money back? The company goal was to collect large revenue, and if we could successfully do that without having to fear documentation collection on every charge, then we were profitable. The more I looked, the more I understood, and the more I realized we must be *very* profitable. There was a lot going on that I still didn't understand.

Days turned in to weeks, which turned in to months as I continued working the financial counseling position. I thought it would never end, and the pile of problems I encountered seemed to grow almost as rapidly as my stomach did. Five months passed and I pressed Janine each week to find out when the position would be filled. Her response of "soon" now sounded like a bad tune.

When the stress of maintaining this demanding position became too much, a temporary solution was offered. I could work four hours upstairs and the remaining four downstairs. This offered limited relief, because patients now found their way down to my second floor office bringing their complaints. Several weeks passed before I learned someone had been hired to fill the financial counseling position. However, her manager needed her assistance longer

in her current position. Janine had told them week after week "it was no problem," and at the expense of my health, I was livid!

Pushed to the point of intolerance, Janine was informed I would be placed
on immediate maternity leave via recommendation of my physician if nothing
changed. Results were immediate, but the secrets I had learned from my experience of dealing with financial counseling issues remained with me. I shared
some of what I had learned with a few trusted co-workers and found out they
also knew these billing practices were occurring. Each felt there was nothing
that could be done and feared the repercussions more. I was continually
reminded that if I valued my job, I would remain silent. With the responsibility of a new home and a child on the way, it was frightening and too over-
whelming to say or do anything about it. I would be on maternity leave for six
months soon; something was sure to change while I was away. It had to.

Maternity leave started earlier than expected. The stress of maintaining
work responsibilities of two full-time positions within an eight-hour shift had
taken its toll on me. One more week to go and I would have that long awaited
break. Those last days dragged on. Surprisingly, the training of the new counselor became my responsibility as well. With all that had occurred through the
years, I should have expected this. During my final days of training, I found
myself doing a countdown. At least for a while I would be free from this place,
free from the pressures, and free from the corruptions I held secret.

The time away was wonderful, and as the days passed I found life as a
mother overpowering any negative work reminders. Periodically, I checked in
with co-workers to see how things were progressing and was continuously
told, "nothing has changed." Refusing to believe this, I convinced myself
something must have, but upon my return, I was in for a surprise. Everything
felt familiar, perhaps declining more. There seemed to be no hope in sight,
and with the startling news that John had suffered another heart attack there
was nothing else to do but wait.

A staff meeting was called immediately and everyone was informed of
John's health status. According to his doctors, he was expected to make a full
recovery, but bed rest would be required over the next several weeks. Paul
would temporarily handle his work responsibilities. I was worried about him a
great deal, but also saddened, because I knew there was no one in the upper
management arena I felt comfortable enough with to turn to for support. This
truly felt like a dead end.

In the meantime, we were instructed to proceed as usual with our daily
business activities. She spoke with urgency as she stressed *now* more than ever

the importance of processing claims and billing accurately and consistently. Everything was to be timely, and on occasion we might have to take certain measures to ensure we had met required deadlines. Firmly gripping the papers she held in her hand, Janine's tone turned crisp. *"We will meet them."* Everyone exchanged glances; there was nothing to say. The message was clear, and it had been relayed for too many years.

To our surprise, we learned that guests would be joining us for this meeting. Dr. Welch and Dr. Johnson were expected within twenty minutes. They were coming to discuss upcoming changes with the way they wanted their billings processed, as well as a few problems they had encountered. We were warned to listen closely, take notes, and our staff would meet briefly afterwards for feedback. Three rapid knocks on the door stopped Janine in midsentence. Putting on her professional face and a broad grin, she opened the door, welcoming the doctors and inviting them to occupy two vacant seats I had failed to notice. Waiting, Mark, Megan, and I locked eyes briefly as if to say, "This should be good."

Listening, it became evident that most physicians were feeling the burden of receiving documentation requests.

Dr. Welch commenced the meeting, reminding us that he understood the importance of chart documentation. He wanted us to understand that his primary concern was providing patients with the best care possible. Everyone agreed. With the way things appeared to be going in the department, I was thrilled to hear this remained a priority. They felt tremendous stress with the slow pace of getting some charges processed. This comment had become all too familiar. Dr. Johnson added his comments by reminding the staff how hard physicians at the hospital worked and the fact they should be compensated accordingly. *We should all be so fortunate*, I thought. Dr. Welch ended their discussion with "If these charges are taking too long to get through, that affects our wallets."

Janine jumped in before he could speak another word. "We have just briefly discussed this issue."

I wondered what she meant by "discussed." We hadn't discussed anything; she had done all the talking.

"We are implementing some new practices that will provide improved billing timeliness," Janine continued. I could tell from the smile that now graced Dr. Welch's lips that he was pleased by her words.

A few coordinators shifted in their chairs. The rumblings many had expressed recently about billing volumes were well known amongst the staff.

Everyone was pushing their limits, and it had become clear some of the billing responsibilities handled by one coordinator for various departments needed two people: medicine, neurosurgery, general surgery…The department budget wasn't able to currently handle the hiring of additional personnel, so work would have to be divided. Whoever had lighter workloads would be asked to take on additional responsibilities. Looking around the room at my co-workers, I knew everyone would make sure it was obvious they were busy because it was too much to handle—taking on additional work responsibilities.

"Kissing up" was what we saw now. Janine wanted to make sure everything appeared to be running smoothly. Give the doctors what they want, cause no conflict, and always appear as if we are in control. That was the way the game was played. We couldn't run the risk of any complaints leaving our room and reaching corporate. Dr. Johnson presented his last few comments, and to the astonishment of the staff, Lisa Rogers, a five-year employee of the company, raised her hand to ask a question. All eyes turned in her direction, staring, waiting in anticipation of what she was about to ask.

Dr. Johnson made a swift motion with his left hand, indicating he was finished speaking and the floor was hers. Flipping through a notebook she had resting on her lap, Lisa quickly located the page she was seeking. Using her right index finger, she ran her finger midway down the page and came to an immediate halt.

Lisa's question pertained to documenting *new procedures*. Janine adjusted her business jacket and shifted slightly; her discomfort was evident.

I had always found Lisa impressive, because she was a woman who knew her job, came in each day prepared to do it, required limited management guidance, and didn't cause problems. She was easily approachable and supportive of less-experienced medical billers. The recent shuffling of work responsibilities had involved Lisa with billing for Orthopedics and Neurosurgery, departments still new to her. Today, she wanted information, and we sensed someone was going to have to provide a sufficient response. At the moment, her confidence was reminiscent of Tracey, whom we all still missed.

"I've recently started doing some billing for Orthopedics and Neurosurgery," she commenced…" Lisa had noticed problems with the coding. Her eyes didn't look at Janine, but remained directed towards the doctors. Procedures were being performed, yet there was not an acceptable code in the CPT book that clearly defined what had been done in the operating room. Sometimes physicians would list codes they wanted used on the billing sheets and there were errors. During those times, Lisa stated, it was often pertinent that she speak to a physician for clarification. She reported her technique of calling the physician, leaving a message with the secretary, and following up with a documentation request via the hospital mail system. If there wasn't a response, Lisa reported that she would wait, because she wanted to ensure that she was adequately selecting the proper code. Then she posed the question I couldn't wait to hear the answer to. "Are you going to have a problem with this sort of time delay?" With that said, Lisa paused, gazed around the room, accepting the appreciative smiles of support she received. Mark sat in the corner with a grimace propped comfortably upon his face.

Having been silent for the past ten minutes, Dr. Welch was the first to speak. He stated his appreciation of the feedback and was understanding of the frustration and concern voiced. Dr. Johnson was in agreement. Each felt too many documentation requests were a distraction, and was time consuming. The final solution came when the decision was made to contact them if we were at an absolute loss. They would assist as much as possible to ensure we could do our job as well. Dr. Johnson continued and brought up an important topic: staff training. He wanted to make sure the staff was consistently updated with changes in medical billing practices, coding exemptions, medical terminology usage, etc. They knew we all worked together, but counted on our organization as the experts in charge of billing. They didn't feel they should have to tell us how to do our jobs. We were expected to be fully trained and already know how to do it. There would be exceptions, but each argued that their involvement should be limited.

"How often do you all attend billing and health care seminars?" Dr. Johnson inquired. Instantaneously, the room went silent, and only the chirping of a bird nestled within a bush outside our office window was heard.

As if awakening from a daze, Janine volunteered to check and see when the next seminar would occur and inform them at a later date. It was obvious everyone was uncomfortable now. She had successfully disregarded his question. Practices had changed so abruptly within the company during the past few years, attending seminars was now limited to a few select individuals. I couldn't remember the last time any of the professional fee coordinators were able to participate in outside educational opportunities. Janine would attend seminars of her choice with a friend and a fellow company manager; prior to going, she would check to see if there were any questions staff members had. If there were, she would make note of this and promise to return with answers. Hearing the details of happenings while at these seminars, it was clear they had more "free time," often involving a little shopping on the side, rather than educational opportunities. Many profee coordinators resented this and voiced their frustrations amongst themselves.

Despite not having their question answered, Dr. Welch and Dr. Johnson appeared pleased with Janine's concern about upcoming seminars. Motioning for the doctors to follow her, the three departed, walking across the hall towards her office to continue their discussion. I wondered what she had to say that was so private. As the staff began rearranging their chairs to designated spaces, the meeting was adjourned. Everything was about to return back to normal, or so we thought.

Within a week, another staff meeting was called. Everyone assembled, and it was evident from their facial expressions that there was tremendous curiosity in the air. This time there was no statistical review or review of staff goals. Janine went straight to the point.

"We have had to make some changes within the company to maintain goals and standards expected by the hospital physicians. Our timeliness was always a priority, but also we had to be in compliance with rules established by Medicare, Medicaid…To help us meet these goals, we have created a new position. I have the job description here, and if anyone is interested, please feel free to apply. We want to have the position filled by the end of the month and we hope someone from in-house will fill it. I can think of a few qualified candidates myself," she continued, glancing around the room. "For those of you already at pro-fee coordinator status, this is not a big advancement. It is pretty much straight across the board, but if you are interested in a change in work responsibilities or learning something new, you might want to consider this option. Does anyone have any questions?" No one did, and the meeting ended almost as quickly as it had begun. A few of us glanced at the board, but no one seemed too interested. The position seemed like too much of a headache for a company that, from the inside, appeared to be headed toward a cliff.

Compliance Officer

It was only a matter of weeks before the compliance officer, Carrie Watkins, was in place. She was to be the answer to many of the issues the company was addressing. Her major priority would be to ensure that the company was staying within the boundaries established as medical billing laws. Employees were assured her expertise would remove many pressures already experienced by workers. Carrie was a well-known, likeable, six-year employee who used her skills, as well as her charms to advance up the corporate ladder. Having previously worked for Louise and Janine, there was no question about her capabilities in succeeding in this position. After scheduling meeting times with employees at the University Hospital branch of our organization, I, too, had no doubt about her potential. Perhaps now something would change when others discovered we weren't following the guidelines, as we should. I could only hope.

When it was time for me to sit with Carrie and explain my job responsibilities, I did so proudly. Despite what was going on, I was well compensated, there had never been any company layoffs, my medical benefits were being paid in full, the retirement plan was terrific, and I enjoyed my basic job responsibilities. Carrie was in her position full throttle. Our department scheduled the commencement of an audit to begin the following month. This time Carrie was at the reins.

Carrie asked numerous questions as she rummaged through a patient file. The documented report was there, but the signature was missing. "These are not truly valid without the signature," she commented.

Tell me something I don't already know, I thought. I watched as she began furiously writing on her yellow legal-sized pad. The distortion in her eyebrows showed her displeasure with the evident inadequate documentation she found. While the hours passed, her questions increased, as did the pile of charts she set aside to discuss with Janine. Wheeling the medical cart across the hall with her pile stacked high, I slyly buzzed Mark's intercom.

He answered comically, indicating he knew who was on the other end. I reminded him it could be anyone buzzing him, but he had seen the easily recognizable intercom number. Panic was getting the best of me lately.

"Keep your ears open. Something's about to go down," I whispered.

"Gotcha," he replied.

Thrusting down the receiver, our conversation ended. Returning to work, I gently massaged the tension headache I felt developing. Lately I had felt tired constantly. There were so many thoughts racing through my mind, I felt unsure of the strange sensations I was experiencing. I forced myself to focus on the claim forms on my desk. They were due soon. The thought of not meeting my two-week deadline for processing these requests concerned me.

The shrill tone of the telephone ringing interrupted my personal massage as I gently tilted my head from side to side. The tightening in my shoulders lessened and I answered the telephone with my usual greeting. "University Physicians. May I help you?" Surprised to hear John's fragile voice on the other end of the line, I hesitated, unsure of what to say next. We exchanged several minutes of friendly conversation before his tone took a serious approach. The questions now focused on Carrie and her new position.

"She's doing wonderful," I exclaimed, sounding as cheerful as possible. There was really nothing I could complain about; I wouldn't have anyway. What good would it do? My conversation was briefly interrupted by the *screech* of a medical cart in desperate need of oil. Carrie had just returned to our office, minus the files she had taken across the hall, and our eyes crossed in a quick glance as she greeted me with a friendly smile. I looked for signs to indicate her mood, but nothing showed. Her gaze told me she was curious who I was talking to. I seized the opportunity.

"Here she is right now," I said. Before John could say another word I motioned for Carrie to pick up the line and placed my call on hold. Listening to their casual conversation, it became apparent they had established a comfortable working relationship. This was good to hear; perhaps she would be successful at convincing corporate to make necessary changes where others had failed. Returning to my duties, I wondered how much time would pass before Mark made his way across the hall. Megan glanced discretely in my direction. Despite Carrie's friendliness, we reminded ourselves that she was a manager, and we remained careful what we said around her. It was important that she make discoveries on her own. She appeared relaxed, and it wasn't long before we noted sometimes she was almost too relaxed. It soon became obvious she had fallen easily into the "management clique."

The "management clique" consisted of about four individuals who discussed all the work issues, as well as the gossip going on at the various company locations. Carrie, Janine, Audrey—a fellow manager, and Monica Parsons were members. Monica was the only one in the group who was non-management. However, her friendly relationship with Janine kept her apprise of all the inside scoops. This was common knowledge and infuriating to fellow staff members. Because of my work location in the central office rather than a separate upper floor, I was exposed to a great deal of knowledge, but I remained tight-lipped on information I was willing to share—personal or otherwise. The risk of where that information could end up was too great.

Stepping up to the Plate

Carrie began meeting with physicians and UWP corporate management on a regular basis. Our staff members were not always privy to what occurred during these meetings because sporadic information was offered, and that was only occasionally. At times Carrie returned to our office, making sarcastic comments about the physicians and their controlling ways. Our suggestions were requested in the best approach to dealing with certain physicians and the issues we felt were priority. If that information was valuable, who knew? But soon Carrie's carefree spirit seemed to pass along to the physicians. One day as I observed her and Dr. Walters, Medicine department, engrossed in conversation, their laughter told me they were comfortable with each other.

The commanding façade of our compliance officer displayed cracks within months, and problems I believed would be tackled were ignored. It became obvious Carrie was in a battle with job responsibilities and wanted to create a steady appearance of superiority. Several employees noted her workdays within our office were spent gossiping on the telephone with friends or family. She made no attempts to hide this fact. Her vocalizing continued to reveal her hopes for our organization. Silently, many of us hoped her goals would become real. If so, the environment would become respectful again. I feared this would never happen after becoming witness to a heated argument between Carrie, Janine and Stephen.

Our three management representatives became embroiled in a heated discussion involving documentation issues and the extreme to which these problems would be allowed to escalate before they were brought to the attention of John and Paul. To my astonishment, they were willing to continue their discussion, with no concern for Megan and myself seated in the room, hearing everything. Janine wanted problems concerning the hospital kept in-house because she felt she was "capable of keeping things under control." Stephen

50

believed it was important to make John and Paul aware of problems, but still limit the information shared. Carrie was the only one wanting to divulge everything. "Let's tell them the truth. Things are getting out of control here and we must come up with a plan."

Janine's shrieking brought the battle to a momentary halt. Carrie and Stephen appeared surprised by the outburst, as were Megan and I. I knew from this response that Janine felt cornered. Taking a moment to regain her composure, she commenced again.

Janine had major concerns about what information was passed along and the portrayal of situations within the department. John and Paul were known for comparing workers and management between the two hospitals. Janine feared acquiring the appearance that she couldn't handle problems in house. Carrie's facial expression showed understanding, but her raised hand expressed disapproval.

Carrie felt upper management should be allowed to help us, and everything should be thrown on the table before things escalated out of control. Everyone knew if the physicians became unhappy they would start complaining, and that would cause major problems.

Stephen agreed with Carrie but felt the information shared should be limited and continued to press his point. After what seemed like hours, Janine's temper reached a boiling point and there was no more hiding anything. She had a point to make and they were about to hear it.

"Listen here, you two," she snapped. Her left foot tapped repeatedly while her right finger darted back and forth between Stephen and Carrie. "At the end of the day you're not stuck dealing with the doctors or John and Paul; it is *my ass* on the line taking the heat. *Neither one of you will say anything.* We will work together to take care of things and *if* all else fails and we are *forced* to say something, then we will." As she stood with her eyes racing back and forth, it was evident to all in that room that she meant business. Turning my head slightly to the left, I glanced over at Megan working quietly at her desk. Locking eyes, she quickly looked away, signaling her discomfort with all she had heard. A footstep disrupted the moment, and after taking three steps into the room Mark glanced around, sensing his timing was bad.

Looking around, he politely excused himself, turned and left. No one said a word. I didn't look at him, but I could feel his gaze. Mark knew I would fill him in later on any pertinent information. The heated exchange ended. I wondered if they believed an understanding had been reached. Discomfort was felt in my limbs. There used to be a time when I could voice my concerns to Stephen, but no more. His job promotion changed him drastically, and as far as I could see, he had become one of them. Our conversations were now limited to work and current events.

Returning several minutes later, Carrie plopped into her seat and began working as if nothing had transpired.

She spoke briefly about her frustrations with the turn of events in the office. No one offered a comment. Realizing that she wasn't going to receive an answer, she dropped this line of questioning. The next day, and every day after that, I noticed a change between Janine and Carrie. Janine turned on the charm, and I believe it was her way of ensuring that Carrie did exactly as requested. Whatever the goal, it appeared to be working. The two soon reconciled and began having lunches together. Preparing to return to the main office to complete additional responsibilities, Carrie left a list of patient names with us, asking if we would pull the charts for her and set them aside for the following Friday. She needed to examine them. She had learned the Medicare auditors would be arriving within the next few weeks. All too familiar with the tension about to invade our offices, I knew the days ahead wouldn't be much fun.

Learning the Truth

Carrie returned a week later, as promised, to a large stack of files awaiting her. Laying a checklist out on her temporary desk, she began working her way through each file, asking questions along the way. This time she was more detailed than before because she knew professional auditors would be rechecking them soon. Whatever was found could affect the company tremendously and that kept the pressure on her. She had been hired to protect us—to make sure everything was legitimate. Many documented reports were missing and she asked repeatedly what we did to acquire them. She appeared startled to learn all the places she would have to go to obtain copies. After checking with Janine, some of those responsibilities to acquire the documentation were passed along to us to speed up the process, as usual. During her daily routine, Carrie found the documentation problems more frustrating. After trying unsuccessfully on numerous occasions to acquire needed paperwork, she passed along the major problems to Janine. It became Janine's problem to decide the best course of action, since several involved surgical procedures totaling over $5,000.00 per procedure.

Janine agreed to give each problem personal attention later that day. Carrie looked unconvinced, but gladly passed along the paper work, even if her escape from it would be only temporary. Janine took the files back to her office and returned a short time later.

"Here you go," Janine said proudly.

Carrie's questioning look was met with Janine's look of deception. Looking at the first few, Carrie was amazed to see what we had known all along. The physician's name had been typed onto the report.

Carrie explained that signatures were still needed. Convincingly, Janine elaborated by stating that documentation was acceptable "as long as the report contained the physician's name."

Janine pointed and Carrie looked on, realizing the reports did contain the appropriate physician name.

"*It is there, isn't it?*" Janine practically shouted.

Turning to leave the room, Carrie looked after her in amazement. I wondered what she would do with the information she was learning about our departmental billing practices. After all, she was our compliance officer.

For a couple of weeks the routine was the same as it had been so many other times. Rush, seek, any problems, fix immediately. All too quickly, time ran out. Auditors were coming the following day and everything was in place and ready to go. This time Carrie was concerned if she had done her job well enough to impress upper management. Staff members working in room C214 just wanted this audit over. This time there were two auditors that would be seated in our UWP offices. One auditor would work in our room and the other in Janine's area. News traveled quickly through the grapevine, and the pressure was on.

Things were underway as Ms. Parker and Ms. Stevenson introduced themselves to the staff. They had been instructed to check in with the staff in our office prior to commencing the audit. Observing the charts on the back table, they knew they had reached the appropriate destination.

"Good morning, ladies," I said cheerfully, sounding like a greeting committee. My desk faced the door and was the first one noticed upon entering the room, so I felt obligated to speak. I introduced my co-workers and asked Barbara and Megan if they could help get things arranged for Ms. Parker. Leading Ms. Stevenson across the way, the heavy pounding of her pumps in the hallway sounded forceful. Introducing her to Janine, I left and happily returned to my desk just in time to answer the ringing telephone. It was Carrie calling and verifying the arrival of the auditors.

I informed her "they've arrived," but felt uncomfortable speaking about someone sitting so closely to me. Carrie requested a call if there were any problems.

"Sure," I responded, attempting to conceal my sarcasm.

The audit was now in full swing.

Glancing towards Ms. Parker, I tried to remember how many audits I had sat in on through the years. 6,7,8…too numerous to recount. Reminiscing further, I couldn't remember ever hearing negative results surface after an audit. Despite having had the tension filled preparation time, I believed UWP would prevail as a winner once more this time. Our organization had mastered the documentation game and we were all forced to play our parts if we wanted to maintain employment. Sitting next to Ms. Parker, I felt tremendous guilt. Who was willing to testify about the injustices being committed? The last conversation I had with John about documentation still echoed in my mind.

"No one else has ever said anything to me about documentation problems."

Did he suspect I was exaggerating? I wondered. I had approached Mark once about using his name as another person witnessing major billing errors, but he wasn't ready to do it then. I needed to try again. I desperately needed him to be ready, because I couldn't handle much more of this environment.

"Are you OK, Swannee?" Turning, my eyes were met by the concerned gaze of Ms. Parker. Apparently she had called my name several times and noticed that I appeared to be lost in deep thought. Embarrassed, I politely thanked her for her concern. She had a question about a chart. Being the closest to her, I stepped forward and by the looks on Megan and Barbara's faces I could feel their relief. Ms. Parker had flipped through a chart several times but failed to see a report. She wanted me to double-check her observations.

Taking the file and her scribbled notes, I returned to my desk in search of the report. The first time through I didn't see it, and I flipped through it again. The report wasn't there. Hesitating, I gave her my final verdict. "No, I don't see it anywhere in the file."

She thanked me and picked up the chart once more.

"You're welcome." I smiled. Making additional notes on her pad, Ms. Parker tossed the chart in a separate pile and went on to the next one. In the end I wondered what it would all mean. When Janine and I had a private moment I informed her of the missing report. She smiled, unconcerned, and I wondered how she could remain so confident.

"There won't be many like that at all in the pile. Remember they have all been checked. Everything cannot appear perfect." Winking, she headed down the hallway with her hair swinging in a rhythmic motion. Replaying her words, I understood her message. There would be a few minor mishaps within the files because *it had been done intentionally.*

The auditors finished their chart reviews in eight days. Through our mini-conversations I found Ms. Parker to be extremely pleasant and as we said our goodbyes, her words chilled me. "I have never found another hospital with documentation this good. I wish all of our audits could go this smoothly." Waving at her, I bit my inner lip until it hurt slightly. That was the only way I could prevent its trembling.

We found ourselves returning to our usual routines almost overnight after the audit ended. The environment was more relaxed, and when Janine disappeared to her management meetings, things were all smiles. Some co-workers from upper floors that limited their visits to known times of Janine's absence stayed and chatted. Each co-worker, sharing common problems in their billing area, feared retaliation if they spoke about documentation issues. What could we do? Bills to pay, families to support, and an unstable economy—no one was willing to risk losing their employment, benefits, and retirement funds. There was a code of silence amongst staff members. Seeing that I had failed to get a response from upper management only heightened their hesitation to speak. I couldn't blame them. On more than one occasion John had promised to discuss problems with Paul, but nothing more was ever said. In fact, I had recently begun to feel as if John was intentionally avoiding me. If not for the conversations I had with Mark, Megan, Barbara and a few others, I don't know what I would have done. Friends I had spoken to outside of my work environment didn't understand the full extent and overwhelming burden and guilt I carried daily. I was unsure how much longer I would submit to this intimidating environment.

Health Problems

I had recently noted an increased trembling in Barbara's hands and wondered if it had anything to do with the environment. Casually mentioning it one afternoon, her squirming made it apparent it was a topic she was uncomfortable discussing. Apologizing for the personal intrusion, I reminded her that Megan and I would assist her in meeting required deadlines. Politely offering thanks, she assured us there were no problems. The end of the week proved otherwise; after meeting with Janine, she returned looking worried.

Glancing in her direction, Megan began questioning her, trying to determine if everything was all right.

"Yes," Barbara replied in a tone barely audible. People at the main office had been complaining about her slow work habits. She explained she was doing the best she could. We agreed. This had been an extremely busy time for all of us.

"Just say the word *if you need us,*" I reiterated. Barbara shook her head, appearing grateful. Somehow, I knew she was too proud to ask for help. Megan and I casually began removing work from Barbara's pile and processing the reports ourselves. Once finished, they were placed in her completed pile and she never knew she had the help. We watched for months at the end of the day as Barbara carefully slipped a stack of claim forms that needed coding and the current ICD9 coding book into her bag. As she waved goodbye, each of us looked on, knowing she had a long evening of work ahead of her.

Disaster struck when Barbara fell ill one evening and wasn't able to come in to work the following day. Calls from our company patient relations department came in regarding claim forms, and when Mark hurriedly raced into our office, having overheard Janine's conversation about some problems with Barbara, I knew there was trouble. *Rat ta tat, rat ta ta...* she was coming. Throwing open the copier, Mark flipped a chart onto the screen and pressed start, pretending to obtain needed information. Luckily, Janine paid him little attention and I could almost hear him exhale.

Janine was searching for Barbara's work. Glaring at me, Janine awaited my response as to where she should look for it.

"I believe it is all on top there," I lied, pointing to her completed workbox. For the past weeks, Barbara had been placing work in her desk and locking it at the end of each day. She knew, as we all did, our desks were searched after hours, but she still hoped her backlog volume could be concealed. Unfortunately, Janine had easy access to our desks. I felt a lump form in my throat as she pulled keys from her pocket. There was nothing any of us could do to stop her. We looked on as she easily slid a bright gold key into the lock *Click!* Hearing the dragging sound of the center drawer and the rattling of the lower drawers opening, she was in. We knew what was coming; looking up, Mark had quietly exited. I wanted to run, and looking at the door I could tell Megan had similar thoughts.

"What the hell?" Janine didn't even finish her thought. The only thing heard was the swish of page after page being turned. She pulled out stack after stack of papers from Barbara's desk. *Bam!* Her fists pounded the desk. She slammed the drawers of the desk shut and stomped out of the room like a hurricane blowing through a small town. Then there was silence.

Barbara returned a day later, and for the second time within two weeks she found herself locked behind closed doors in Janine's office. Thirty minutes later she returned to the office, speechless. The bright redness in her cheeks said it all. Before providing us with the details, we could figure out pretty much what had occurred. Her job was in jeopardy and she desperately needed it.

When Mark, Megan, and I had an opportunity to talk, we filled him in on what had transpired with Barbara's situation. I read a lot in his eyes.

Knowing Barbara was a private person, it was obvious she hadn't been feeling well lately. Mark felt they should "give her a break." Speaking with conviction, his compassion was evident. Unsure how much Janine had shared about Barbara's current health situation with John, I still believed he should have some understanding considering his own health issues. In the end, we all agreed we couldn't allow the mistreatment of Barbara, but we needed a plan. We believed if we pushed too hard that might cause added problems.

Janine entered the room, causing us to jump and informing us we had better return to work. Trying to explain that we were chatting momentarily, we were clearly reminded that we were not paid to stand around having conversations.

"If you don't like your jobs, remember anyone can come off the streets and do this work." This statement had become a familiar annoyance.

We all knew this wasn't true, but having heard this repeatedly, our self-esteem was deteriorating. We had somehow been berated into believing this. Now, as we slowly moved back towards our desks like a herd of sheep, I knew we truly did believe it.

Carrie's Role

"Surprise!" The sound of a familiar voice caused us to look up. It was Carrie. We were surprised to see her at the hospital. Usually there was some sort of advance warning that she was coming. She began talking politely, explaining that she, Paul, and John were there for a meeting. No one really cared what she was doing there. Departmental morale was low. No one felt valued. Things were slipping through the cracks, billing requirements were overlooked, and massive cover-ups were occurring. What happened to the workplace I once enjoyed? I no longer wanted to be a part of it all. From the moment I had hired on, my words to John were "I will remain here as long as I am happy." I had worked for the company since my teen years, believed I couldn't go elsewhere, and didn't feel happy about my job. Deep down, I knew Janine was wrong for preaching the negativity she did to us, and one day I would prove it to her. For now, I would continue using Marcella's office and the office of a few other co-workers fortunate enough to have their own workspace when I needed a temporary break. It was my only escape.

Carrie was searching for Janine. Today, the ring of her voice was annoying.

"She's in her office," I replied, no longer caring about showing enthusiasm.

Carrie felt Janine might want to attend their meeting, since it involved the Neurosurgery department.

"Perhaps." I was direct—tired of having small conversations when it was convenient and treated like a peon at other times.

Janine appeared on cue, seemingly pleased at Carrie's presence. Quickly filling her in on our conversation, she invited Janine to the meeting. I could see in her eyes she didn't care to go, but felt, as management, she should. *Why wasn't John or Paul here extending the invitation?* I wondered.

Surprisingly, Darcy was being included. This would give her an opportunity to meet some Neurosurgeons. She presented this thought in a questioning tone. Carrie offered her support and approval. I found the interaction of the two amusing. Janine had seniority within the company; however, during the past year Carrie had nestled herself into a superior management role. Management was impressed by her and grasped each word she said like a lifeline. Amazing! With Darcy in tow, the three headed down the hallway. A minute later I heard Janine returning. What was the problem now?

Handing me a postcard with a desert on the cover, I gazed at it curiously. It was a postcard from Lorraine, and she was visiting family in Las Vegas. Reading her message, I smiled for what felt like the first time that day.

"I will visit you all soon," it read. Silently, I prayed she would.

Mark appeared, wanting to know what was going on. I began discussing how unhappy I had become recently. There was too much stuff going on. Turning serious, Mark reminded me I did have one major advantage; I didn't have to share an office with Janine. Laughing at his point offered temporary relief.

Lately Janine had resorted to watching Mark like a bulldog. I held my hands up, pretending to growl. We both chuckled and fell silent once more.

Mark stressed that something needed to change soon to improve our work environment.

John had been talked to more than once, without yielding any results, but Mark believed another tactic should be attempted. I didn't understand his meaning and I certainly didn't feel powerful. Mark felt proof should be gathered that proved what was going on within the company, then it should be given to the right people.

"And just who are the right people?" I asked, leaning forward just as Stephen entered. His timing was uncanny.

As he questioned us about what was going on, an immediate diversion came to mind. Handing him the postcard, I explained that it was from Lorraine. Reading through her brief but friendly message, Stephen smiled.

"I miss her." His response surprised me. He had changed so much lately I wasn't sure he was the same person I had met years before. His behavior reminded me of Janine, focused on working and having as few problems as possible. The last time I attempted to discuss a work problem with him, he went off on a wild tangent about how unappreciative the staff was and the fact that they should limit the complaining. And now having his own office, he was free from many of the burdens he had once faced on a daily basis. More importantly, how quickly he had forgotten about all that was occurring around him. Mark gave me a look that seemed to say, "Don't worry," and politely excused himself. Lately, he and Stephen had clashed on a couple of billing issues. I believed their problems stemmed from Stephen feeling left out of the "information loop." Denying this, Stephen proclaimed his problems with Mark revolved around his lax work ethics. I decided to remain neutral.

Darcy, along with Janine following steps behind her, returned from their meeting shortly after noon. Their appearances displayed little energy, and by their limited conversation I suspected all wasn't well. Smiling at Darcy as she collected papers from her mailbox, I gave her a slight wave as she left. Checking her own mailbox and retrieving messages, Janine left moments later.

Darcy and Janine began working together on billing issues. We began to notice, as suspected, that Darcy had limited comprehension of coding for the more complex procedures occurring in the Neurosurgery department. Surprisingly, this appeared to be of little concern to Janine. I learned through other co-workers this was because Janine's sole concern remained keeping the position filled. Several others had been approached about taking on that billing service, but there was so much protest nothing was ever done about it. Everyone was hesitant to deal with the "arrogant" neurosurgeons they had seen. With everyone professing to have too much work, Janine was left to deal with Darcy and all that entailed. As I listened to the rumblings of many, I realized this deal was serving a purpose for Janine: keep a warm body in position and everything else will be dealt with.

It didn't help to know profee coordinators were no longer attending coding meetings or seminars. I couldn't remember the last time I had seen anyone go. Carrie continued to go to those available, and as she returned she made the decision on whether or not she felt particular information was worth sharing. Often co-workers were told, "There was nothing new introduced." Repeated requests to attend classes were denied because of the expense. The company now found it more valuable to have Carrie's presence solely. This infuriated many of our profees. Many staff members felt that since Carrie wasn't a coder, she didn't have the right to make decisions about what information they should be privy to. I agreed. That was about to be substantiated by the physicians.

The handsomely dressed Dr. Myers arrived at our office door, requesting to enter. I recognized him as a long time, well-respected neurosurgeon. Motioning for him to come in, Barbara offered assistance. He was looking for Darcy. Explaining that her office was across the hall, Barbara arose to guide him there. However, before they could leave the room, Darcy entered, placing a pile of charts on the cart. Her eyes widened and her facial expression appeared distorted upon eyeing Dr. Myers.

Barbara explained intently that she was just about to bring Dr. Meyers to her office to talk to her. Darcy's facial expression looked fearful. I headed towards my desk as Darcy asked to use an empty corner of the room to talk to the doctor.

"Sure," we replied in unison. Ignoring our puzzled expressions, she pulled two chairs to the corner. Why work in a small, stuffy, corner when she had her own desk across the way? It made no sense, but as their conversation began to unfold, I understood. Listening to her stammer through coding explanations made me feel sorry for her. I wished there was something I could do to help her.

Dr. Meyers was concerned about Darcy's selection of codes. He felt the ones she had selected for a particular patient didn't properly describe the procedure at all. Plus, the fee should have been billed as a partial fee. Dr. Meyers had only performed a portion of the procedure. This billing was a major mess, and Darcy sat there, appearing lost while the conversation continued. Unable to grasp her wording, she looked back and forth between the papers that were resting on her knee. Shifting slightly, Megan's chair made a screeching sound, causing them both to look around. With tears welling up in her eyes, Darcy began to speak, offering the only explanation she could think of.

Many apologies were vocalized and Darcy promised to speak with her manager as soon as she returned. Dr. Meyers appeared stunned that was all being offered. He continued questioning Darcy, and for the first time his irritation was evident. This was unacceptable. Darcy was just too unsure to proceed with any attempts at reconciliation herself.

"Please check into this and get back to me ASAP. These billing problems are occurring *too much*," and with this stern warning, Dr. Meyers vacated the room, without looking back. Darcy sat for a few minutes in silence, looking at the papers she held, until the sound of someone else entering the room made her look.

Janine was back, announcing it as if she had won a prize. I don't believe any of us cared that she had been gone. Sensing something was askew, Janine looked from one face to the other. No one offered any explanations. Looking concerned, Janine demanded to know what was going on. Without a word and to my surprise, Darcy got up, allowing her tears to flow freely, and left the room. Looking after her, Janine turned back, facing us with a look of panic.

I offered the shortest explanation possible while Barbara listened. "Dr. Myers was here with some questions. Darcy had a difficult time answering them, and he wasn't very happy." I stopped, determining the two of them could discuss the rest privately. Janine stood erect. She understood. Darcy was in a job she didn't understand. She was drowning, and everyone knew it.

Turning, Janine mumbled something about calling Carrie. I don't believe she realized that she was thinking out loud.

That afternoon Carrie arrived, and as suspected, they excused themselves for a meeting. They never said where they were going, but we all knew. My intercom buzzed; it was Mark.

"They're heading to Neurosurgery to try and fix this mess."

"I suspected," I replied, limiting my comments. It wasn't fair the way Darcy was being treated. Mark's next comments addressed the promise that he would one day find a way to fix this mess.

Hanging up the telephone, I clung to his words. He sounded so serious that somewhere in my heart his words rang true.

Carrie and Janine returned two hours later, looking content. I would have given anything to have heard what they said during the meeting. I knew from past experiences that everything was probably made to appear as if it were Darcy's fault. Shortly after this incident I noticed a change with the Neurosurgery billing. Several of the department physicians were familiar with coding policies and began presenting precoded log sheets to Darcy for billing. Some called other UWP profees for assistance with their billing. Darcy's mood relaxed, and it was evident that she appreciated the changes. Janine appeared receptive to the idea of physicians doing some coding and justified the situation by explaining that if some of the physicians wanted to do their own coding, we would let them.

I wondered about this practice, and during one visit when Darcy and I went to obtain a needed signature for a billing, a last minute coding change made me uneasy. As we prepared to leave, the physician wanted to make a change on the billing fee sheet. With a few scribbles, it was done. "Insurances pay better for this code, and it's only an extra cut up this way," he offered, motioning with his hand. Appearing pleased with his knowledge and coding skills, he handed the paper to Darcy. Her hand trembled. She was instructed to enter the charge into the billing system that day and she agreed, just like an obedient child. I looked on, saying nothing.

Where's my Money?

The holidays were fast approaching, and the physicians were beginning to charge more. Janine was losing control and everything seemed chaotic. Common physician complaints about UWP circulated the hospital, and several were outspoken about their frustrations. Many were beginning to question our competence. At times, being part of the organization became embarrassing. They wanted their billings done timely and properly, and when it wasn't being done, they continued to step in. They were allowed to, so why not? Paul and John were well aware of many of the practices by now and didn't appear to be too concerned. The rest of us allowed fear to silence us. There was so much at stake. Occasionally, I wondered how to prove our accusations. If the people in charge were not willing to listen, who could we turn to?

Dave Rawlings, union steward, seemed like a good place for me. We had known each other for a year and a half. I joined the union, much to Janine's surprise. She confronted me in a threatening manner about my decision to do so. I was frightened, but with numerous changes occurring in the workplace, my membership felt like added security.

Listening carefully to my words, Dave offered feedback on what I should do about some of the treatment employees were experiencing within the organization. I wasn't comfortable revealing everything I knew about billing and documentation practices—not just yet. Janine entered the room to photocopy several files, but appeared to be listening to my conversation. I chose my words carefully and sensing the change Dave suspected someone was nearby. Ending my conversation, Janine reminded the staff of our time limits on the telephone. Quickly explaining that I was speaking to a fellow UWP employee, my explanation was disregarded; I knew then I had best be careful or suffer her wrath.

Despite the tension, the department was thrilled to learn we had once again achieved our predetermined billing goals and would receive an end-of-the-year bonus. Everyone had worked hard and we deserved it. A month later, with the actual checks in hand, our excitement turned to laughter. The amount was just barely two hundred dollars. No one could believe it, and it was evident from the look upon the faces of staff members that everyone was expecting more.

"This isn't even enough to buy my groceries," one complained. I looked on, disappointed as well. Tearing her envelope open, Monica looked at the dollar amount and grinned. We all knew she felt the same way, but because of her friendship with Janine she wouldn't comment. As everyone stood around, chatting and looking at their bonus checks, Janine managed to slip into the room unnoticed and hear some of the criticism.

"You should all appreciate the fact that you got a bonus. The managers don't even get that," Janine explained. I was surprised to hear this. I assumed they did. When Janine shared this information, she failed to realize that Carrie voluntarily released management information to staff members, and her comments told another story. We soon learned they did receive bonuses, indeed.

Two more days and we would have a couple of days off for the holiday. I could barely wait to have some free time. The profees raced around, attempting to enter the last of their billings into the computer system before the holiday. As I worked some last minute problems, the telephone rang consistently. With Barbara and Megan already responding to the first lines, I answered the third line when it rang for the second time.

"University Physicians." I waited. It was Carrie looking for Janine, who had just run down the hall to the restroom. Carrie wanted to discuss problems with Neurosurgery billing codes. The physicians were writing codes that didn't exist on the fee sheet. I promised to relay the message, but I knew some sections of it must be omitted. This would only mean more problems for Darcy, and I almost dreaded leaving the message. In Janine's opinion, if Darcy knew how to do her job they wouldn't have all these problems. I also knew Janine wouldn't be happy at the prospect of us knowing more than she felt we should. It had become known that she prided herself in "keeping us in our place," a fact Carrie had failed to learn. With the ballpoint pen in my hand, I carefully constructed a note. It read: "Carrie called, needs to discuss neurosurgery codes." She could find out the specifics on her own. Taping the note to her in-box, I silently said a prayer for Darcy.

The displeasure physicians experienced because of billing issues eventually reached the corporate office, and several calls were received from John and Paul. Each gentleman sounded serious as they requested to speak to Janine at her earliest convience. Both gentlemen arrived at the hospital for a meeting with Janine and Darcy several days later. Their presence within our office was limited to a brief "Hello." Despite being pleasant, both gentlemen had demonstrated the words "Everything is flowing smoothly," which was their primary concern. In a matter of minutes, they had left the room heading next door. Janine rang my intercom.

"Darcy and I are in a meeting; please hold our calls."

"I will."

With their meeting in full swing, Mark made his way to my office. He knew this was a good time to visit, because he was safe from any watchful eyes. His timing was ideal also, because I was the only in the office and we could talk freely. Plopping onto the chair next to my desk, Mark placed a charge-out slip on my desk. We chuckled as he explained that this would be our cover in the event someone entered the room and saw us sitting and talking. Perfect! Glancing at the slip, I realized it was a chart medical records claimed was signed out to me anyway.

Running his fingers through his black-feathered hair, Mark questioned me about how I was holding up. I looked around slowly before I spoke.

"This is difficult, because I like many aspects of my job and my co-workers, but I need to get out. I have worked here so long now the thought of leaving scares me."

"You're smart, Swannee," Mark replied. "You can always find a job somewhere else." We laughed aloud as I reminded him that was not what Janine had to say about it. We both realized it was being done to demean us, and unfortunately we were allowing it to work. I wanted an immediate solution about what else could be done. Mark expressed the opinion that we hadn't spoken to the right person yet to get anything done, but until he could tell me who the right person was, I wasn't going to be satisfied. I noticed something different in his tone; this time there seemed to be so much conviction. I believed him, and I was clinging to that belief with everything that I had.

That afternoon I learned my backup support was needed on the financial counseling position again. I prayed that Mark would erupt with an idea. I could feel my tension brewing as I realized it was one thing to know deception was occurring, but to live the lie, talk to the victims face to face, and pretend like everything was all right was something else. This was taking things to another level—something I wasn't prepared to do. Gripping my clipboard and yellow tablet, I headed towards the third floor financial counseling department. My mind was racing. Walking down what felt like the hallway of misery, for the first time I allowed myself to set my burdens free and say the words I had needed to say for years but had feared: "I am going to quit this job."

I was stuck once more and ended up, surprisingly, spending most of my week working upstairs, providing assistance to hospital patients. This time around I found it even more draining and couldn't wait for it to be over. The one advantage was that Mark and my other co-worker friends were able to stop by for friendly, casual conversation without being placed under a microscope or having our visits timed. During my breaks and lunch hour that week I spent my time searching the classified ads in the newspaper and checking the bulletin board in the hospital's first floor personnel office. Day by day, I was becoming more determined.

Ringggg! The sound of the telephone distracted me from the insurance paperwork I was matching up for a patient.

"Good morning, financial counseling. May I help you?"

It was Mark calling. He wanted to meet me in the main lobby in fifteen minutes.

His mysteriousness captivated me and I wondered what he had in mind. Perhaps we could end the year with a little excitement. Little did I know at the time that his suggestion would be so daring.

Setting the Trap

"You want to do *what?*" I almost shouted.

"Keep your voice down, Swannee," Mark reminded me.

"I'm sorry, but I just didn't realize my friend was so crazy," I whispered. Mark had always had a carefree attitude, but collecting proof of documentation problems to be used later was risky. What if he got caught? What if someone suspected me of helping him? I was terrified of this risk, and there was too much at stake. Sure, I was already searching for a new job, but I definitely didn't want to be *fired* before I found another one. Listening to additional details, I realized that he was serious and ready to start gathering information immediately. I felt myself perspiring profusely. Reluctantly, I agreed to help. We agreed to put the plan into place as soon as I began working at my desk again. He would do the work and all I had to do was provide the extra set of eyes to help keep watch. Sworn to secrecy, I vowed to remain silent about what was about to transpire within the walls of UWP.

I had stood alone previously in my battle to expose the truth, and I had wasted too much time. Now I had help. Replaying everything in my mind, I knew there was no other way. We shook hands. *This had to be done.*

Returning to the financial counseling desk, I found myself easily distracted by thoughts of what was about to occur. A company paper trail was about to get started. One after another, patients flowed in with reoccurring problems, and a glimpse at their patient accounts on the computer showed nothing had changed from before. The primary difference was that now I could read patient accounts, and I understood company codes, insurance codes, transactions, occasional write-offs, and the ability to see where monies were held and applied, double insurance payments that were kept—it was all there. Everything was clear. I felt disgusted. Politely excusing myself, I informed the hospital financial counselor in the next cubicle that I needed to run to the restroom. Within minutes I entered the small restroom, and to my amazement the usually crowded room was vacant. Feeling flushed, my stomach churned viciously. I felt sick. Stepping into the cramped stall, my body convulsed, releasing all that it held.

Returning to my temporary work area, I sensed fellow employees looking at me.

Maria, a petite Filipino woman in her late fifties, asked if I was feeling okay. Her small hands gently caressed my back and her face showed concern.

"I'm fine, thanks for asking. It must have been something I ate," I lied. Guiding me towards the cubicle, she told me to tap on the wall if there was anything I needed. I agreed, appreciative of her kindness. Turning, I was startled to find a couple who looked to be in their mid-forties waiting on me. Taking a deep breath, I propped a smile on my face and offered assistance. Introducing themselves as the Wilson's, I quickly searched my memory bank, recalling a conversation I had had with the wife via telephone the previous day. They were participants in the hospital's Invitro Fertilization program. Having collected payments from numerous patients for these treatments, I knew the expense involved. The wife was the first to speak. They had paid for their hospital portion of the procedure earlier, but had a balance of $5000.00 still owed to the physicians. Making room on the desk, I informed them that the payment could be taken within minutes. Opening her purse and pulling out her wallet, Mrs. Wilson handed me three credit cards.

"I don't know how much room is left, but charge what you can on each one. We've tried this two times before. *We just want a baby.*"

Taking the cards from her, I looked into her eyes, took a deep breath, and wondered if the charges she was paying were legitimate.

Megan grinned broadly when I returned to my office. It felt terrific to be back at my own desk and away from the pressures of the financial counseling position. Barbara and Megan admitted to missing me. I was happy to see them both as well, and I began to relax. Rubbing the soreness in my neck, I sat down at my desk, looking to see what work duties had been neglected while I had been working upstairs. Barbara and Megan had been nice enough to open my new mail and process some reports for me. This kept my workflow going. I was appreciative, because Barbara was still facing her own health battles.

Stephen made a brief appearance to say "Hello," to everyone and perform his daily mailbox check. Sometimes it saddened me that I couldn't open up to him. He was no longer trustworthy, and I had learned through a series of incidents that my feelings were valid. However, there was no reason we couldn't remain professional. With the formalities complete and Stephen's minimal contribution to the conversation, he departed and the rest of us went back to work.

Mark entered the room, handed me a piece of paper, and left abruptly. Glancing downward, I noticed a small yellow post it slip stuck to the front. It had two words written on it: "This afternoon." The message was clear. There was no turning back. Paperwork collection was about to begin.

Buzz! My intercom rang, and Janine asked me to come to her office. I was nervous because through the years I had learned that most of the times when you were summoned to her office, it meant trouble. Walking slowly towards her room, I reminded myself that she knew nothing about what was to come; there was no way she could. Motioning for me to sit down, she left her office door open, which made me uncomfortable. This was a common tactic of hers that she used to prevent any argument from staff members. Knowing someone else was hearing the conversation limited the chances for that. She began speaking without even bothering to say "hello."

Janine held my recently-approved vacation request in her hand. I wondered what the problem was, since I had more than enough time available to cover the time off. Imagine my horror when she explained she wanted me to cancel my vacation time and allow financial counselor Shirley to have the time off. It was explained that I had had time off several months ago. I don't know what difference that should've made. Within minutes, it all became clear. Shirley had threatened to quit her job if she wasn't given the time off. My temperature was boiling, but I managed to pull myself together.

"Sure, no problem," I managed to say in the sweetest tone possible.

"You will?" she almost shouted. I nodded my head, yes. My jaw muscles tightened.

The relief she felt from my response showed on her face like a brightly lit bulb. Movement in the background reminded me that others were sitting behind me. I was accustomed to having "open" meetings, and wasn't fazed by the reminder. Expressionless, I waited for the discussion to continue. To my surprise, Janine turned her back to me and began dialing her telephone—a sure sign this brief meeting was over. Arising, I turned, preparing to leave, taunted by her laughter ringing in the background.

"Shirley, everything is fine. You can have your time off." I needed a few minutes alone and took a brief walk down the hall before returning to my desk. Everyone looked at me as I entered the room, without saying a word.

Somehow, I was sure they knew what had happened. Information had always traveled fast between the two offices. Taking my seat, I looked down and noticed a note neatly taped on the center of my desk. My name was written in Janine's easily recognizable handwriting. Opening it, I read the following message:

"Thank you for forfeiting your vacation time for December 26th and 27th. Christmas is an important time for being with family and I appreciate your understanding."

My blood boiled. The letter seemed to imply I didn't have plans with my family during the holiday. I knew this note was just a written reminder for me to come to work the day after Christmas and cover her ass. I resented it, and as I folded the note into quarters and slipped it into my purse, I smiled. I wasn't too worried, because I knew by the time that date rolled around Janine would be holding a note from me: my resignation.

Later, during a talk with Mark, he informed me, as suspected, that he had overheard our entire conversation. His gentle words put me at ease and I promised to move ahead and support him, without dwelling too much on Janine.

He had been steadily collecting proof of documentation errors. I was excited about the prospect of having some possible results from the injustices I knew had been committed. Still, I remained fearful and cautious. If he were caught, what would happen? Mark asked what time I would be leaving that afternoon. He looked pleased when I responded with "my usual time: 3:00 p.m." Earlier that day he had overheard Janine on the telephone. She would be leaving for the corporate office today at 1:00 p.m. That would give him plenty of time to rummage through the recycle bin.

My palms began to sweat at the thought of this and it took a minute before I could speak. I needed to be sure that he was prepared for what was about to commence. We both knew that once this started, there would be no turning back. Looking in his eyes, I noticed an assertiveness and determination I had never seen before. It was agreed that after Janine's departure, he would begin his collection process. I would buzz him if I sensed anyone was heading his way. The buzz would give him enough time to toss stuff into his drawer. He wasn't worried about Darcy, because she didn't pay much attention to what Mark was doing most of the time anyway. I agreed with his plan and didn't view Darcy as a threat, either. Hours later, I watched Janine stroll down the hallway, leaving for "a meeting." Ten minutes later my intercom buzzed, signaling it was time to put things into full swing. I was ready.

Things couldn't have worked out better. Darcy poked her head into our office shortly after Janine left and told me she was heading to the upper floors to retrieve some files. Mark had the office next door to himself. I sat, talking to my officemates, trying not to think about what was happening. I could tell no one because the risk was too great. Within the hour he rang, indicating he was finished.

"Find anything?" I asked, choosing my words carefully so no one else would be aware of what we were discussing. He had found a few things, but nothing considered major. Mark was convinced that more things would become available later in the week.

"Be careful," I stressed.

"Now you know I always am," he laughed. "Besides, what is she going to do to me?" he joked. I didn't know the answer to that question.

I often wondered if Janine would ever have the courage to fire Mark. He was unconvinced she would, because she was "all mouth." It was agreed that Mark would check the recycle bins every chance he got, and if we viewed anything suspicious we would notify each other.

Monica and Stephen entered the office, demanding to know if they had missed anything exciting. I was sure Janine had asked them to do their usual spot checks and verify that everyone was working and where they were supposed to be. Monica's casual questions about others only verified my suspicions. Stephen immediately began inquiring about the whereabouts of Mark. "He's working next door," I reported.

"Who are you kidding?" Stephen asked, almost laughing.

"Well, I don't see you working too hard," I shot back. I had lost a lot of respect for him. Stephen informed the group he could be reached at his desk if anyone needed anything. I chuckled silently.

That's a first, I thought. Lately he had been known for roaming the halls, chatting with the ladies. I didn't care what he was doing as long as he stayed away from our work area.

Monica waved goodbye and was on her way as well. I suppose she didn't find too much of interest here, because her visit was short. Janine didn't return that afternoon, which wasn't surprising. She had become known for "calling it a day" after her meetings.

As the day came to a close, I had one final thought I needed to bring to Mark's attention. Where would he keep the information he collected from the recycle bins? It was risky to keep the paperwork in his desk. He assured me he would collect the items, place them in a special folder, and take them home.

"What are you going to do with all the information once you have it?" I asked.

"I don't know," he laughed. "Maybe I'll call the FBI and turn it in."

I laughed at this thought myself.

Visitor from the Past

The next day was busier than ever. I didn't know what had happened at Janine's meeting the previous day, but something had shifted her into high gear. She spent most of the day behind closed doors in her office, and when she ventured out into our office we heard mumblings about unprocessed billing and claim forms.

The familiar chant of the importance of staying on top of our billings filled the office. When Janine talked about comparisons made between the accuracy and timeliness of our medical staff and the UWP staff located in Harborview Medical Center, everything became clear. There was a sort of competition going on. Over the past few years, Janine had become extremely close with Audrey, her counterpart at Harborview, but she always considered herself the better manager. Any success Audrey had, Janine needed to prove she was better. Having heard repeatedly about the wonderful work Audrey did and the limited problems she had with staff and billing issues made it clear that this was getting under Janine's skin. Also, having Carrie impressed by Audrey's work only made Janine feel more threatened. As John and Paul began demanding quicker response time and solutions to ongoing problems, Janine appeared more out of control. She had extra monies in her budget and had asked for assistance with the Nephrology, Neurosurgery, and Medicine billings. It had been approved. Loretta was returning to help out. I was thrilled.

Loretta had recently returned to town and was available to help out for a short time. To Janine, it provided the perfect solution: bringing in someone familiar with the environment to help out and it wouldn't require any training. The following week when Loretta made her way back to the offices she had called home for over ten years, I was the first to race to her, embracing her warmly. In her face I saw someone familiar, trusting, and to whom I desperately needed to talk.

Talk we did, as soon as we had some free time. It didn't take long for Loretta to fall back into sync with the billing practices. However, it was strange to know she was no longer in charge. How I wished she were. I knew things would have been so different. Situated at a desk near Mark, she began working her way through the charts, and it wasn't long before she approached me with a question.

One Friday afternoon she asked if I could look over some papers she held in her hand. They were from the Nephrology Department. It appeared the doctor listed had no involvement with the kidney dialysis treatment, yet the fee sheet she had indicated that she should bill for it as if he had. Loretta wanted to know what was going on, and I gathered my thoughts carefully before speaking. I had heard this comment too many times. Quickly explaining that that was how the billings were processed now, I will never forget her stunned expression. She recognized that things had changed a great deal while she had been gone. Janine entered the room shortly afterwards and Loretta wasted no time in posing her question to her.

Explaining the situation carefully to Janine, Loretta made sure no details were omitted. Loretta stressed the fact that the billing needed to be changed since the information was inaccurate.

Janine explained that it was acceptable and billings were now handled differently.

"*You do?*" Loretta questioned as her tone escalated. Looking at Janine, she awaited further explanation. None was offered.

"It's been done this way for a while. Just bill it." Returning the paperwork to her, Janine turned, preparing to leave.

"Is this even legal?" Loretta asked finally. To that, Janine said nothing.

Loretta did as instructed, but after she and I had an opportunity to talk over coffee one day she began to get the big picture of how much things had really changed. She commented that things were not like that when she was the manager. I knew this all too well. She wanted to know what had happened to an organization that was once so well-respected and when the change occurred. It had been this way for so long I didn't know where to begin.

When I told her the way employees were being intimidated, verbally abused, overly stressed, she was speechless. Loretta believed John and Paul might offer a solution. I shook my head no. The disappointment in her face was revealed. Loretta sat, motionless, as I continued to offer further explanations. After hearing of my numerous attempts to warn John about problems and his assurance of relaying information to Paul, but nothing had happened, it was obvious that Loretta was hurt. Loretta remained for several months, processing work using the new method. Our eyes met during her final day of work for the department, and my sadness remained evident. I could tell she felt joy in seeing her former employees, but she now found that the integrity of the company had been compromised.

Mark had successfully collected numerous pages of paperwork, despite Loretta's presence, for the past few months. He knew he needed to acquire more and at a quicker pace. Inviting me for lunch that afternoon, I sensed he had something else on his mind. As he began eating his burger, I learned what his next step would be. He would begin to come in to the office in the evenings and on the weekend. Processing the information slowly, I asked, through a mouthful of food, if he was far behind.

"No, Swannee. I am coming because I need more time to collect the papers from the recycle bin. It is getting too risky during the day." I now understood his reasoning, but I was uncomfortable with this information. I reminded Mark that Janine came in to process work occasionally on the weekends. I wondered what he would say if they encountered each other.

"You are going to help me make sure that doesn't happen," he commented. I looked on questioningly.

Mark would let me know when he planned to come in. If I learned that Janine planned to do so on the same day, I was to tell him. I understood. Mark was moving ahead full force.

We had both noticed more papers being thrust into the recycle bin over the past several days. Janine had gone into "spring cleaning mode." Recently she had been overheard on the telephone requesting special "recycle pick-ups." What this was all about remained unclear, but we assumed something important must be concealed within the box. Mark needed to ensure that he searched the recycle box before the recycle staff got their hands on it. He did. It wasn't long before *he hit pay dirt.*

In a short period of time Mark had managed to collect volumes of paperwork which showed inaccurate and inconsistent billings, residents or technicians performing work on patients and the attending physician charging, proof of codes being changed for higher reimbursement (upcoding), and pages clearly indicating that John and Paul were well aware of many of the inconsistencies occurring because their signatures were on the correspondence memos retrieved from the bin. The paperwork proved surprising, but Mark proceeded, convinced he had only just scratched the surface. His belief was that if

injustices were going to be proven, there needed to be enough paper work verifying the accusations. We were battling years of injustice.

Mark had began to notice that Janine appeared tense. His radar detected
something was up. He knew it might not be easy to determine what was causing it, but he remained determined. I wasn't sure what he had in mind. He
believed some secrets could be found in her in-box. Mark decided to start
checking her mail. I was horrified. This meant pushing things even further
than I expected. There was nothing for me to say. The fierceness in his face
showed there was no stopping him. The following afternoon he began doing
just that. The office next door was empty for a short time and as he appeared
in my office for a few minutes, a double tap on the door let me know it was
time. I listened carefully for sounds indicating someone was heading towards
our office and cringed at the risk he was taking. Mark successfully collected
more damaging memos that helped me understand why John and Paul did
nothing about many of the problems. They were already aware of a great deal
of the problems. That afternoon as Mark and I talked, he handed a stack of
papers to me that made everything clear. John and Paul had made things clear
to Janine. "Give the doctors what they want." It was right there in front of my
face. I had never felt so betrayed.

Several days later, I received the call I had been praying for. A manager
from a local aerospace company called regarding an interview. Responding
immediately, an interview was arranged and a week later I had an offer on the
table. I now had a way out of UWP. Janine was wrong; other employers found
us worthy of hiring, and I soon had a typewritten offer in my hand proving
just that. It was time to resign.

Sharing my wonderful news with a few of my fellow co-workers, I watched
as they looked on in disbelief. We had all talked about how unhappy we were
for long periods, but somehow no one believed anyone would ever do anything
about it. I had reached the breaking point and was willing to risk everything.
As Mark entered the room, aware of my plans, Barbara walked up to him asking him to convince me to stay. His response will stay with me forever.

"None of us want her to go, but we don't want her to stay here and be
unhappy. She has to go, and this has nothing to do with our friendship."
Through tears, Barbara nodded her head, while Megan looked on. I felt tremendous guilt, knowing they would be left behind.

I worried about Mark and what would happen to him. Shrugging it off, he
smiled. I could see sadness in his eyes. There was no one remaining within the

department that he was close to, either. Assuring me that he would be fine, he vowed to continue on with the struggle.

I questioned Mark, wanting to know how much longer he planned to work for the company. Ruffling his newly trimmed hair, he said he was uncertain, but estimated perhaps another year or two. I gasped, not believing what I had just heard.

With the small talk out of the way, he reminded me there was another major task that required my attention. "Go in there and tell Janine you're about to get the hell out of here." To hear Mark say those words so freely was empowering, but somehow I still feared Janine's response.

After an hour of reviewing what I was going to say to her, I finally pushed Janine's intercom number and waited for her to answer. Surprisingly, she sounded cheerful. Tightening my grasp on the telephone receiver and wiggling my fingers nervously, I managed to find the right words to say.

"Hi, Janine. When you have a minute I need to come over and talk to you about something." I was caught off guard when she immediately invited me to come over. I anticipated having more time to prepare my last speech, but there was no turning back.

"I'll be right over," I informed her. Grabbing my neatly typed resignation letter, small notepad and pencil, I was on my way. Why did I grab the pencil? I believe it was to scribble in the event nervousness should overcome me. Barbara and Megan were stapling reports to claim forms as I arose from my chair. Both looked up at me, aware of what was about to happen. I gave them the thumbs up sign, turned and left.

With a vibrant smile resting upon my face, I walked into the office next door. Looking in Mark's direction, I raised my eyebrow slightly as an indication I was about to deliver my message. His wide grin showed he could hardly wait to see her reaction. I did a double knock on Janine's door and she turned around, instructing me to come in. I did something unusual; I took the initiative and closed her door behind me. I was well aware that she disliked this, and for the first time she looked uncomfortable with me. The power had shifted.

Chatting for a few minutes, it appeared she was going to continue to ramble. I don't know what had gotten into her, but I suspected it was nervousness she felt. Stopping her in mid-sentence, I made a request. "I need to tell you something, Janine, and if I don't go ahead and say it, I may never get it out." Pausing, I began again. "This is very difficult for me, but I am here to give you my resignation." For a moment the room was still, as Janine gazed at me in astonishment, with her mouth agape. Her appearance gave the impression that she thought I was teasing her.

"No, this is for real. I am leaving in two weeks." I released a forced smile. I felt angry—angry because one person had the ability to transform an environment and make it unhappy for so many—but I kept my composure.

Her next question almost brought me to tears. She wanted to know why I was leaving. Gripping the pen I held in my hand, I slowly allowed it to move across the tablet that was resting on my lap. Looking at her, I frowned and said "Because I don't like it here anymore." Appearing dumbfounded, her next statement was even more puzzling. She wanted to be assured that my leaving had nothing to do with her. I couldn't believe her words. Janine professed her sorrow at seeing me go before placing my letter in the center of her desk.

"It was just a number of things, Janine," I explained. Before she could say another word I arose, opened the door and walked out. There was nothing more to say. Hearing the all-too-familiar click of her telephone receiver being picked up, I smiled. This time she was calling to share some news, but I was the one who had defined the terms.

Goodbye UWP

As the door closed behind me, I began walking, unsure of where I was headed. The next thing I knew, I found myself in the financial services area. Shirley was on the telephone with a patient, and when she noticed me sitting there she held up one finger, indicating it would be just another minute. *No problem*, I thought. I had all the time in the world. What's Janine going to do now? Fire me?

Sitting down, I could hardly wait to share my news. Suddenly, I wanted to tell everyone. I hadn't felt this free in a long time. "I just wanted to let you know I turned in my resignation five minutes ago." Shirley froze, and *click*, that beautiful image was sealed in my mind. The news spread like wildfire and I received call after call from people, asking why I was leaving. I was careful with my responses because I wanted to remain professional. John called that afternoon, stunned by the news. "It is time for me to move on," I explained.

Expressing his sorrow about my impending departure, I knew that in his heart he was sincere. He truly was a kind man, and I would forever be grateful for his assistance in helping me acquire my first real job. John invited me to come for an exit interview to discuss any final issues. Glancing around the room, I saw Megan photocopying a stack of medical files and Barbara struggling to meet her deadline. I was going to be gone soon and they would remain, still subjected to the declining environment. They didn't have the liberty to speak their minds without repercussions. I had to do it, not just for my own piece of mind, but also for everyone else within the company that wasn't allowed to have a voice. I agreed to meet with John on my final day. I told Mark about my exit interview plans. He felt this was the time for me to tell John everything. I was ready.

That night I sat down to write what I believed was going to be a brief letter to John about the employment practices at UWP-University Hospital. By the end of the evening it had developed into an eight-page roller coaster letter of my employment history.

Here are a few excerpts from the letter:

> The time has come for me to pursue other adventures in life. Perhaps sooner than planned, but I know in my heart the timing is right. One of the greatest joys of my job during this long work history has been my fellow co-workers and the job itself. From day one I vowed to give my all to any position held within the organization as long as these two factors were applicable. I knew that if either one changed it would be time for me to move on. That time has arrived.

> Every day I go to work I think of the beautiful little girl God has blessed me to have, and all my dreams for her. Trying to raise her to be a strong, proud woman. If I allow myself to repeatedly be treated in the manner that I have over the course of the past several years and being subjected to the mistreatment of others, it would go against everything I believe in—everything I have fought so hard to accomplish.

Court Cafe

> This is not fair. People tell things they feel are safe, but instead, this information is discussed over morning espresso in Court Cafe. I have been a witness to this myself, as have several other workers, and even individuals not working within our department. Part of our staff has been heard more than once being referred to outside of their names by our manager and this angers me. You may expect that from someone else, but not from your leader.

> Profee coordinator Mark Erickson has been preparing himself for over six months with a separate documentation folder that shows evidence of the massive illegal billings that have occurred within the kidney dialysis area. It is terrible. People are frightened by what they know. Even "Louise" has questioned the way these billings are occurring. The response of "Oh, this is the way the billings have

always been handled, so just pick a doctor and bill it" is no longer acceptable. From the profee coordinator's point of view, this is wrong, especially when you are billing for a physician and have documentation that proves he was on vacation during the time you have billed for him. It is becoming a moral issue for many profee coordinators. Now, since not only are the businesses being sought out in audits, but so are the coders.

Many want to speak the words that I have chosen to, but they cannot, because for now they still must work under "Janine," and for that I sympathize with them.

Take the time to care.

I am no longer willing to put up with particular occurrences at University Hospital (UWP). Now I need to bring some important points to the attention of those who can bring about a change for the workers remaining.

These events had brought me to today. My final day of employment with the University Physicians had arrived. Glancing around the room one last time, I allowed myself to take in the scenery that had become "family" during the past thirteen years. The limp plant leaning against the rear wall, continuously growing for years despite being virtually ignored. The creaking, metal desks with jamming drawers I had struggled with, the newly delivered photocopier that was already jamming when copying…We should have kept the last one and saved the money, I thought and chuckled. And, the memories of growing, learning, and embracing new friendships seemed to tackle the negative, at least for the moment. A lone tear fell, which I immediately wiped away before anyone could see it. There was no time for that. Janine had already taken too much from me and I wasn't about to let her see my pain. There were a few brief goodbyes, kisses, friendly exchanges, and promises to maintain friendships shared. It was time to go. Lifting my box, I heard the *clink* of my coffee cups. The sound seemed to indicate a send-off. With a final wave, I turned and headed towards the door. Proceeding down the hall, I felt my feet moving faster and faster as I remained focused only on the straight path in front of me. Down and out the second floor emergency entrance. The opening of the electronic doors seemed to signal freedom. I stepped out into the chill of the afternoon air and inhaled. Refusing to look back, I moved on, feeling a freedom that had escaped me for years. It was time to move on, but I had one task lying in my path.

Exposing UWP

The elevator doors opened as I moved forward, carefully navigating my way to the front desk.

"Mr. Reed is expecting you," I was told.

Following the receptionist, I found myself walking farther and farther to the back of the room. Passing desk after desk, I could feel eyes peering at me—familiar faces I had come to recognize through the years. Their expressions seemed to say, "We know why you are here." My face gave away nothing! I moved on. I had something to say, and John and Paul were going to hear it. Entering John's office, I found Paul had been called away to a last-minute meeting and it would just be John and me. John's blinds remained open, allowing other staff members to peer in as they walked by. Carrie walked by within the first half hour I had arrived and could be seen reaching for a phone almost immediately. I guessed who she was calling, but was unconcerned. No one could hurt me now.

Delving right to the point, I spilled my soul, summarizing all that had happened through the years, giving examples where needed and pleading for a change for the remaining employees. Explaining my concern for these employees, I stressed how fearful they were about speaking up. Having spoken privately to Mark before leaving, he said he was willing to speak up about what he knew. I believed, since Nephrology was his billing area and major billing inconsistencies were occurring, his testimony would be powerful. John appeared horrified, and this caught me slightly off guard. Maybe he didn't understand as much about what was going on as I thought he did. He trusted Janine, too, and she had failed him, I reasoned. As he looked me straight in the eye, his glare seemed to pierce the core of my soul. Neither one of us blinked as he promised that Janine would "never be allowed to treat employees the way she has been, never!" With tears flowing freely, I sat across from John, trembling. I didn't care who saw me. I was hurting. Ninety minutes later I stood up, preparing to leave.

John reiterated how much I would be missed within the organization. Extending my hand to him, I thanked him politely. I truly did appreciate the opportunity he had given me and would never forget it. Clutching my resignation in his hand, John promised to keep its contents between us, but to discuss problems with Janine, effective immediately. Thanking him once more, I smiled, satisfied that its contents would be kept private. Why should Janine be given the opportunity to read it and deny everything? There was nothing more left to say. I was finished with UWP, or so I thought.

"How are you doing, you traitor?" Mark was calling and teasing me about my newfound freedom. It was terrific hearing his voice. I missed him. I could hardly wait to hear the details of John's scolding of Janine. Wondering what else he had done to her, I waited anxiously. I knew she had gotten what she deserved.

"Swannee," he began. I was growing impatient and urged him on. Detecting something in Mark's tone, I fell silent. It was then that Mark explained that John had immediately come down indeed to see Janine. Mark continued on, detailing what had occurred next; Janine and John were overheard laughing at me and my resignation letter.

"What do you mean?" my tone elevated. Janine *never* saw my letter.

"Oh, but she did," Mark explained. "John brought it down here the following work day and showed it to her." I became infuriated, shouting into the phone. I couldn't believe it. How dare he? He promised me! He promised! John had also taken Janine to lunch. I didn't know what to say. I pressed on, wanting to know if John had discussed billing discrepancies with Mark. Mark explained that John had assured him he would look into billing issues and instantly informed Janine what Mark was complaining about. Janine was now riding Mark's ass daily, angered that he opened his mouth. I couldn't believe it.

"I'm sorry, Mark. I failed, and I tried so hard."

"Don't worry, Swannee. I'll take care of them. I promise."

I knew Mark was still collecting paperwork and had a good-sized stack of papers he had collected and photocopied stored at his home, but at this point it all seemed useless. What difference would it make, anyway? I had to move on with my life, and that is what I did.

UWP gets Busted

Four years had passed since I last walked out the door of University Hospital. Cuddling my beautiful four-month-old second baby daughter in my arms I was happy once more, and all that I had previously experienced seemed like a bad memory. There were times that particular situations or sights would trigger some negative memories of UWP, but they were becoming minimal, and I was hoping to keep it that way. As Mark and I talked monthly on the telephone about UWP happenings, I was happy to have departed when I did, especially upon realizing that nothing had changed. How he still managed to survive the place, I couldn't understand.

One April afternoon, as I sat giving my baby her afternoon feeding, a local KOMO television newscaster captured my attention with her breaking news report...

"University Physicians, also known as UWP, is being investigated for fraudulent medical billings said to be totaling in the millions..."

"Oh my gosh!" I screamed into the stillness of my home. I began to tremble. Did I hear right? I had been waiting for this moment for over seven years. I had to call Mark. Reluctant to call the UWP offices, I left him a message on his home answering machine. I could barely think straight the remainder of the day. As I sat on the couch, trying to decide who to call, the telephone rang. Lunging forth like a boa, I wrapped the receiver in my hand and tried to calm my breathing so I wouldn't sound overly excited.

It was my former co-worker Stephen, calling to see if I had seen the news that day. I was surprised to hear his voice, because we hadn't spoken very often since I had resigned.

"We were raided," he began, without giving me time to respond.

"What?" I practically screamed. My infant daughter wriggled with a start. Stroking her back to comfort her, I listened to the details.

"I was in the office with Janine, using the computers, when all of a sudden the FBI showed up." The thought of the FBI made me shake. "They asked for Janine by name. She identified herself and they told all of us to get up and step away from the computers and not to move our hands. They didn't want anyone attempting to delete files. We did as instructed. Janine asked what was going on and why. They said a whistleblower had turned them over for fraudulent billing. Janine was furious and totally caught off guard. They began taking computers, disks, files from Medical Records, and they even *searched my office*." I was so stunned I could barely speak, trying to visualize the scenario.

Asking Stephen who the whistleblower was, I awaited his response. I believed I already knew the answer, but wanted his thoughts. He quickly explained that he and Janine figured it was Mark. I sounded shocked and asked him to explain why. Stephen's response caught me off guard.

"Because he is lazy and this has him written all over it." I reminded Stephen he shouldn't refer to Mark in this manner because it could just as easily have been someone else. Naming off a list of my former co-workers, Stephen explained why everyone except Mark could be excluded. I wasn't positive it was Mark at this point, and even if I were, I wouldn't have said so. Stephen had changed so much; I was reluctant to share anything with him.

"I need to give you a name and telephone number," Stephen explained. UWP had retained an attorney for their employees, present and former.

"Why?" I asked.

"In case you are approached or subpoenaed; the attorney can help you get immunity." This was too much for me to process. Grabbing a pen and paper, I quickly wrote down the name and number of the attorney he rattled off. Why Stephen thought I would want to use an attorney hired by UWP, I was unsure. I thought to myself that they should fear all the information I had stored away. Telephoning my husband at his office, I quickly reiterated what had happened and all I had learned so far.

"Do you have a suit that fits?" he quipped.

"What do you mean?" I questioned, puzzled by this unusual response.

"You want to make sure you have a nice suit that fits properly when the FBI comes asking for your help." I sat on the other end of the telephone, laughing at the thought.

Diiinnngg Dong! The sound of the doorbell ringing interrupted the peacefulness of my Monday morning. My husband was still in bed, and I shouted upstairs, letting him know I would get the door and wondering who it could be. Opening the door slightly, I peered through the bars of the screen door at the statuesque female standing on the other side. Instantly noticing the brief-case and papers in her hand, I prepared to tell her I wasn't interested in what she was selling. She began to speak. Her first two questions captivated me.

After a friendly greeting, I was startled to be referred to by my first name. I nodded my head yes while rising to an erect position. Who was this? She wanted to know if I knew Mark Erickson and had I previously worked for UWP. My head was spinning to hear someone standing at my door and say-ing those haunting letters: UWP.

"Yes to both of your questions. Mark and I are good friends and I used to work for UWP." Reaching towards her pocket, she opened what appeared to be a black leather wallet and flashed a professional-looking badge with a gold shield that sparkled brilliantly like a freshly waxed table. My eyes fixated on its beauty.

"I'm Tory Briggs with the FBI," she said.

My body shook slightly, stunned by what she had just revealed. In a soft tone, she requested permission to come in and discuss my employment and experiences at UWP. Remembering that my husband was upstairs made me feel more comfortable. I opened the door and welcomed her into my home. Entering, she carefully slipped her business card into my hand. Leading her into the family room, I invited her to sit on the couch as I carefully lifted my daughter into my arms. Pulling her close, her infant body gave me feelings of peace and confidence—something I needed if I was going to stroll down memory lane. Opening her notebook, she pulled out a pen and began writing.

Our discussion began with the statement about University Physicians being under investigation for the fraudulent billing of medical procedures. I explained that I had recently learned this information from a local news report. Pausing momentarily, I looked at her, forcing myself not to cry. "I have been waiting for this for years," I continued. "I tried so many times to expose what was going on, but no one would listen."

"That's what we heard," she continued.

My curiosity aroused me. Who did she hear that from? I wanted to know if it was from the whistleblower, and was that Mark. It was then that she explained she was not at liberty to discuss this information during the investi-gation. I understood.

Reaching in her bag once more, she opened a manila folder and pulled out a stack of stapled pages which she handed to me. Looking down, I began reading the first few sentences and looked up instantly. Cringing, I sat there with my mouth agape. My past had returned.

"Do you recognize this?" she asked at last. I still couldn't speak.

"Did you write this, Swannee?" she questioned. Lifting my eyes to meet hers, I searched deep for my voice within. At last it came—scratchy, but there.

"Yes." It was my resignation from five years prior. What was she doing with it? The last I was told, Janine had a copy of it that she was flaunting around.

"Well, Swannee, if you wrote this, I need to tell you, we need your help." I was frightened by her response. My testimony was needed in their case against University Physicians.

"Just tell me when, and I'll be there," I offered with conviction. I then learned it might require that I testify before the grand jury. I sat, stone-faced. This was too much for me to process. I was terrified.

"I'll be there, Agent Briggs,"

She smiled at my response.

The next couple of hours were spent discussing the seriousness of the crime University of Washington Physicians (as they were now calling themselves) was being charged with. I still couldn't believe this was really happening. I had one month before I needed to testify. Agent Briggs explained that a subpoena would be sent as a formality. I understood; everything was perfectly clear. This was truly happening.

One week later a certified letter arrived at my home. Tearing open the envelope, I knew what to expect. However, once I saw the subpoena I felt nauseous. I learned my testimony would occur one week earlier than expected at the United States Federal Courthouse on 5th and Madison, downtown Seattle, 9:00 a.m., before the Grand Jury. Now it was *confirmed*; I had to go before the Grand Jury. I had been trying for years to get the word out, and now I was going to have an audience of listeners.

Attorney General Richard Haskins telephoned me at my home several days later, requesting a time when he, Agent Briggs and myself could meet and prepare for the trial. He carefully explained that he wasn't trying to tell me what to say, but he wanted me to know what areas they planned to cover during the testimony. Agent Briggs had informed him of my nervousness and he did his best to put me at ease. I was instructed to "go and *tell the truth as you know it.*" Our conversation ended on a friendly note, with our agreeing that the two of them would come to my home the following day for a meeting, since I had a small infant to contend with. This time my nervousness subsided tremendously with their friendly greetings. I still wondered how Mark fit into the picture. Our conversation several nights before had left me puzzled. Claiming not to be the whistleblower, I continued to run through my memory of former co-workers, wondering who was. Mr. Haskins and Agent Briggs ignored this topic, and I respected their obligations. As we sat on the couch and began our discussion, I focused on their every word. I now believed I could trust them. I had to. We were on the same side, and fighting for the same thing: justice.

Mr. Haskins observed the droopy eyes of my infant daughter. She was tired and I joked about the rough life she had as a baby. He asked to hold her. Surprised, I agreed. Carefully, I slid my daughter into his arms. He held her gently, with limited movement, over the next hour as our conversation continued. Suddenly, Mr. Haskins turned serious. He had one final, important question I needed to answer. He wanted to know if there was anything from my old personnel file that UWP could dig up, use, or twist to make me appear to be a disgruntled employee.

"There is nothing," I stated forcefully. He needed to be certain.

"I was an outstanding employee, I did my job, I went to work, and I received several promotions, numerous awards..." The thought of that even being a possibility infuriated me. "As a matter of fact, let's just take a look," I offered, rising from the couch. Agent Briggs looked after me, puzzled. Explaining that I had retrieved a copy of my personnel file prior to resigning, their heads swung inward as they glanced at each other. They were welcome to view it. I still remembered the day I requested a copy of the file. Janine gave me a hard time about requesting it, but I knew it was my right to have it. I didn't want to risk something being falsified in it at a later time. Now, more than ever, I was thrilled that I had taken the time to do this.

Moments later, the file was in their hands. Glancing through the papers, their smiles said it all.

"Terrific," Haskins offered. "We're sorry to press you like that, but we had to ask."

I understood. They were only showing me what I could face in front of the grand jury. Drifting into deep thought momentarily, Mr. Haskins noticed my distraction. Leaning forward, he asked if there was anything else I wanted to know. I did have one concern.

"I just want to know if I will run into any former co-workers. There are many I would love to see, but I don't want to take the chance of running in to Janine, John, Paul...That situation would just be too uncomfortable." He understood.

Arrangements had been made for me to be the first witness of the day. I was informed that I might be there for a couple of hours, but there shouldn't be anyone else affiliated with the company there. This response satisfied me and I smiled broadly. Now I was ready.

Testimony Day

The day finally arrived, and as I drove Northbound on Interstate 5, I replayed all the discussions Richard Haskins, Agent Briggs, and I had had over the past weeks. I remembered all I had experienced and prepared myself mentally for some of it being painful to relive. Mounting the last steps towards the United States Federal Courthouse, I carefully opened the door and walked in. A small line had formed and as I read the overhead signs I followed suit, preparing to go through the metal detectors. My breathing intensified as I realized this was the *big* day. Extending my purse out, I was carefully checked before being motioned by the security worker to move forward. Reviewing my paperwork, a guard showed me the elevators that would take me to Courtroom 311.

Walking slowly down the silent, dreary hallway, I watched as the room numbers changed. Soon I stood alone outside my designated room. My instructions were to wait on the bench outside the door and Mr. Haskins would guide me into the courtroom once the grand jury was prepared. Flipping through the pages of the romance novel I had brought for entertainment did little to settle my nerves. I couldn't relax, and watching the ticking minutes on my watch only tightened the pressure within my loins.

An unfamiliar voice rang out from behind me, calling my name. Perhaps Mr. Haskins had sent someone else to greet me.

"Hello, please let me introduce myself. I am Assistant U.S. Attorney, Susan Loitz." Until she said her name, I had almost forgotten that I had been previously told she would be there to meet me. We chatted for a few minutes and I spoke about how awkward it was for me to speak about illegal activities committed by my former employer outside of the company, but I was happy my knowledge would prove beneficial for their case. Listening to details about some of the tactics they had used to ensure documentation was available when needed, I could see disgust in her face. She thanked me for my willingness to come down and share information.

"I tried to share this information with others for years, but no one would listen. No one wanted to hear it," I explained.

Leaning forward, her eyes focused on mine as she assured me "We want to hear it." Our friendly exchange continued as she politely apologized for the lengthy wait. Glancing at my watch, I realized it had been fifty minutes since I first reached the third floor. This was no problem for me; it only provided additional time for me to calm my nerves.

"Just relax and go in there and tell the truth," I was told.

"Yes, ma'am, I will do that."

It was time for her to depart and as we shook hands her words "I will see you in the courtroom" caught me off guard. My eyes bulged as I locked on the friendly-looking round face. I had no idea she would be *in* the courtroom too. I shuddered, wondering who else would be there. Excusing herself, she darted into room 311—my room.

Returning to the bench, I quietly sat down and drifted into my own thoughts. Soon the hallway was filled with silence, but it wasn't long before the clicking of heels could be heard descending upon the floor. A male and female were engrossed in conversation, and when the woman spoke I felt a chill protruding up my spine. It had been five years since I had last heard that voice, but in an instant it seemed like only yesterday. My eyes slowly glided from the black patent leather pumps, to the T length, navy-colored skirt to the unmistakable face belonging to Audrey. The length of her hair was shorter, but I knew from conversations with former co-workers she was still employed by UWP as a manager at Harborview Medical Center. Though she smiled, but said nothing to indicate her recognition of me, her piercing eyes made it apparent. In an instant we both stood facing each other as if in a standoff until the voice of her male companion lured her back in to their conversation. Why was she here during the same time span as I was? I had been assured I wouldn't encounter anyone from UWP, but here she stood. What other surprises awaited me?

I could vaguely overhear their conversation. Audrey was speaking rapidly, and her attentive companion was her attorney, I soon learned. He reviewed a few questions with her as she paced back and forth, chewing her fingernails. Luckily, our reunion lasted only minutes. Suddenly, a smiling Richard Haskins opened the door to room 311. It was time, and as I made my way towards the door, Audrey's voice was heard in the background. "Good luck," she said. I didn't bother to turn around. I didn't need luck; I had the truth on my side.

The friendly exchange of greetings between Mr. Haskins and myself, a few words of encouragement, and one more stop to a small room housing only a table and a few chairs…It was time to make our way into the courtroom.

"Are you ready?" he asked with all the confidence in the world.

"I am as ready as I'm going to be," I replied enthusiastically. Moving forward, it was time.

The doors swung open and I moved on autopilot into the room, my knees weakened momentarily. I had been briefed prior to this day that the grand jury would contain a maximum of 23 jurors, but they had advised me that most days all jurors didn't appear in court. Today must have been unusual, because as I searched the room I could see only one vacant chair. My eyes blinked briefly from the sunlight in the distant window. Why was the courtroom full today? Climbing into the witness box, its smallness generated a moment of claustrophobia. These witness boxes appeared larger on television. Raising my right hand, I was sworn in and ready to begin my testimony.

To my right, Mr. Haskins had risen, prepared to begin questioning. Susan Loitz was seated to his right and offered a comforting smile as my eyes locked on her familiar face. Other than those two, I recognized no one. The questions began and I was asked to introduce myself, spell my full name, repeat it, explain my educational background, employment history with UWP, and what my current employment status was. I easily rambled employment positions held within UWP, as well as the years. It was obvious from the jurors' facial expressions they were impressed that I remembered these details.

The topic quickly turned to company audits, and I sat, allowing myself to reveal the "secrets" I knew. The courtroom appeared stunned and as I glanced at Susan Loitz, she squirmed in her chair. I spoke of physician signature forgery, billings by residents rather than an attending physician, upcoding (using codes that will produce a larger reimbursement from insurance companies)…it all flowed freely.

Mr. Haskins ruffled his papers and brought up the subject of Janine Turner. He didn't look at me too hard. I sensed he knew what that name did to me. Hearing it made me feel like a needle was plunging into my flesh again and again and again. There was nothing I could do to prevent it. This was a painful journey we had to tour. I walked it with determined strength I had never felt before. Every face I gazed into gave me strength that day.

"Did you ever try to expose these incidents you speak of today?" I was asked. Looking around the room once more I talked not to Richard Haskins questioning me, but to the mothers and fathers sitting out there, the sons and daughters and all those who had compassion. I explained the scenario of being verbally abused within an organization, threatened with your job, told you're not worthy, and having your power within the company stripped away, and then you were placed in a weakened state.

"There were former staff members professing their willingness to speak up about situations they knew were occurring, but when the time came they bailed on me. I was left to stand alone. There was no power in that. I was told what they thought I wanted to hear and things never changed. Some employees didn't have as much stress as others because their offices were on other floors and they had their escape."

My explanations continued. "Through the years I watched people being run off from their jobs. One elderly employee was injured severely from a fall and brought to University Hospital; as she was lying on a stretcher, extending her hand to our manager Janine, she was treated like a stranger. Janine said, "Oh, hi," and kept walking. When the employee returned, she was continually pressured about retiring."

"I watched another employee forced to leave because she was willing to work with the physicians to do the best job possible, but she was viewed as being too bossy and threatening. Janine would never get off her back after that."

"Another employee was so stressed out from her mistreatment that she quit her job without turning in a resignation, leaving her family pictures and everything on her desk behind. *I watched this happen time and time again.*"

My eyes felt moist, but I wasn't about to let any tears fall. I had more to say. This courtroom needed to understand.

"I wasn't a disgruntled employee; I was a woman who wanted to be treated with dignity, respect, and compassion. I had feelings; we all did."

Stopping momentarily, I took a deep breath and looked from face to face. Several jurors nodded. *"Do you hear me?"* my internal yearnings were shouting that question. With his facial tone capturing a stern expression, Mr. Haskins strolled towards his desk and reached for a small stack of papers.

He had something to read and I was asked to listen carefully. I was so hyped, I felt ready for anything.

Mr. Haskins continued. "Do you know this author and the context in which this work was used?"

Uncertain where this line of questioning was headed, I promised to do my best and answer his question. With eyes fixated on his lips, I watched as he enunciated each word one by one. Each word projected a powerful force as it burst forth into the openness of the courtroom.

"People are fearful of coming forward."

"Evidence of massive illegal billings."

"Threatening, verbally abusive, unhappy, frightened."

"Please listen and do something."

"Help!"

"I can no longer be a part of UWP."

My emotions were thrust into a painful history that felt incapable of release. I was suffocating, there, in the courtroom for all to see. The ice cool pitchers of water resting on a nearby table made my palates salivate. Spinning, twisting, chaotic—his words dodged past my ears with the speed of a missile. I wanted to escape, and as I looked around with a quivering nose, I bit my lip. Mr. Haskin's pained facial expression showed he disliked doing this, but it was his job. He asked if I was all right.

"I am, thank you," I replied, my breath quickening. Calming myself, I slowly regained my composure. I needed to remind my inner self that I was seated in a place of safety. UWP could not touch me or hurt me. Twisting his arms, Richard Haskins began asking difficult questions. This was difficult because my memories forced me to delve deeper.

"Do you know who wrote those phrases?" Mr. Haskins asked, pacing back and forth in front of the jurors.

"I did," I said shakily, still uncomfortable with the possibility of exposing my emotions to a room full of strangers.

He pressed on, seemingly realizing it would take minimal effort for my feelings to show. I focused on his face; I saw the almond-shaped eyes I was now familiar with, the ones I had begun to trust.

"Relax and speak the truth," my inner voice said. I did, and feelings of over-whelming strength pushed forward. From the bottom of the feet, upward, through the intestinal track, searching for the heart, the voice, the release, and suddenly it was there. I opened my mouth and said "I used those words in my 1995 resignation letter to UWP." At that moment the sense of pain engulfed the room, but the questions moved forward, continuing for two more hours.

It wasn't until I testified that I realized the focus of UWP management bonuses were a big issue as well. I couldn't understand the questioning until I was pressed for added information. Mr. Haskins wanted to know if I was aware that my manager was receiving a bonus. I was. Was she the one that offered this information to me? This required further explanation.

"No, in fact she always denied they were receiving a bonus," I explained. "She always stated we should be happy we were receiving one because they received nothing."

I could tell Mr. Haskins was driving towards a deeper line of questioning.

Trying to grasp the right words, I finally explained, "We had one company manager, Carrie. She was a nice lady, but she talked too much." Laughter was suddenly heard in the courtroom. I looked around and noticed several of the jurors smiling and covering their mouths in an attempt to stifle the noise. It was a light moment. I smiled, too. The laughter sounded wonderful. I continued to speak about Carrie and how she bragged about the excessive dollar amount of their bonuses in comparison to our measly amounts. At the end of this section of questioning, I came away with the impression the company was using some monies they shouldn't have for their bonuses, but this was never said directly, only implied. I was shocked! In all the years I worked for the company I knew there were many things going on, but the thought of something unusual going on with the bonuses I had heard so much bragging about from one individual never crossed my mind. This was startling, especially remembering the small amount of money given to non-management employees.

During the course of three hours, Mr. Haskins along, with two other legal representatives, questioned me. I responded with minimal hesitation as I sat in the witness box that now felt safe, presenting everything I knew about the functions of UWP as I had learned and been exposed to for years. Our topics finished with a discussion about Janine before the tables were turned. Now it was time for the jurors to question me.

I knew this was another aspect of testifying before the grand jury. I had no idea what I would be asked, and I braced myself as one by one questions were presented to me. My speech was firm and audible. The jurors were gentle. I sensed their understanding from the testimony that had already been given. One juror wanted to know what was so intimidating about Janine. Looking at the forty-something, blond-haired female standing before me with an olive colored complexion, I smiled, gathering my thoughts momentarily and allowing my words to flow freely.

"The best way I can explain it to you," I began "is that she was intimidating. If you crossed her path, she never let you forget it and she made it rough for you. It was an uncomfortable feeling, and with your job being dangled over your head you felt forced to comply." She shook her head, showing her under-standing, and offered thanks.

Her final comment before sitting surprised me. "We have heard that a great deal. I believe I understand." I prayed she did.

The questions continued, with the remaining jurors asking questions geared more toward understanding what our job functions were on a daily basis and who participated in what and what they were aware of. Who had control and who made the final decision about things that were done? Explaining clearly and concisely, I felt pleased with how I handled myself on the stand. Also, I had successfully succeeded in doing what I set out to do: be fair and honest.

Addressing the jurors, Mr. Haskins asked for any final questions. An elderly gentleman, wearing a vibrant blue shirt, raised his hand, stating, "I have one final one." My eyes riveted on him. I had come this far, I could handle anything else, but his question caused me a temporary moment of hesitation.

Looking at me, he asked, "You stated earlier you had worked for UWP for 13 years, correct?"

"Yes, that is correct," I responded.

"After all those years, what is the one thing that finally made you say 'I can't take this anymore'?" My response flowed smoothly. I remember the moment when it truly hit me that it was time to leave.

"I was sitting at my work desk one day, working, and my eyes rested on a picture of my daughter. I now have two daughters," I explained to the jurors. "I realized I was raising two individuals who will be tomorrow's women. I thought about how I have always stressed the importance of maintaining integrity, speaking up, and standing up for what you believe in. Then I realized I couldn't teach my children to do that if I wasn't willing to do it for myself." Resting with that thought, I looked directly at him and felt for the first time that he was the one juror who made me feel as if I was going to lose control of my emotions and cry. Dropping my head slightly, I balled my hands into fists, clenching them tightly for support.

"Thank you, Swannee; that will be all."

Looking up, I smiled, allowing my eyes to scan the room one final time. Nearly four hours of my time, and now I was free. At least for now I was.

Exiting the courtroom, I heard footsteps following me and turned to see Richard Haskins. Smiling, I tilted my head to stretch my neck muscles.

"I made it," I said. He was complimentary of how I had handled myself on the stand. I was grateful.

"I just told the truth; that's all I did. I hope they know that." Looking at Mr. Haskins, I felt he was well aware of this. He agreed that the jurors could sense the truth. Saying our goodbyes, he reminded me to call him if I needed anything.

Leaving room 311, I found myself face to face with Audrey once more. I was *stunned* to see her still there. She reviewed my facial expression before speaking.

"How'd it go in there?" she asked. I felt irritated and surprised at her boldness. Feeling as if she was searching for information, I decided to conceal my true feelings.

Exhaling loudly, I managed to speak a few words. "It's tiring; good luck." Excusing myself quickly, I made my way down the hallway, around the corner, and out of her line of vision. However, a knock at my door several days later told me the news of my presence at the courthouse had reached others.

Opening my front door to the sound of double rapid knocks, I was greeted by a male and female, neatly dressed in business attire and carrying paperwork, standing at my front door.

"Swannee?" they asked.

"Yes," I replied, wondering who they were and what they wanted. This felt very déjà vu to me. Introducing themselves as attorneys representing a law firm retained by UWP in a legal dispute, I immediately sensed I wasn't going to like this.

They explained that they were informed I might have some information about the audit and billing practices of the company.

The words "representing UWP" shot past my ears like a boomerang. Why did they want to talk to me? I was just a witness for the FBI. It didn't make sense until they continued to speak.

"Do you know Mark Erickson?" the female asked, shifting her eyeglasses as she spoke.

"Yes, we used to be co-workers," I replied dryly, leaving little for them to read into my comment. She claimed Mark Erickson had mentioned my name.

"Really?" Wrinkling my brow, I looked between them both and stepped back, allowing my screen door to slide back. The mention of Mark's name didn't fit right with what they were saying, but they continued.

They asked if I had been approached for questioning by the FBI. I refused to comment on that question. Recognizing my hesitation, the gentleman jumped into the conversation, assuring me they wanted to hear what I had to say about the company—whether good or bad. "We are on the same side," he offered. By this time they had been standing on my porch with questions for over twenty minutes. I had already declined the offer for them to enter my home and talk. It was clear to me what was going on. They were attempting to find out what I knew *for* UWP. If we were truly on the same side, they would have already known I had testified for the FBI.

Declining their offer once more, I stressed that their line of conversation was painful. I didn't want to do this.

"We can subpoena you," the female representative offered, looking me straight in the eyes. I was mad now.

Looking back at her, I asked if that was the plan the firm had.

"No, I am not saying we are," she offered, detecting that I was becoming defensive. "I am just clarifying that we *can*." I knew what she was saying and had a point I needed to stress that would sum up everything.

"You can subpoena me if you want to, but if you put me on that stand you just *may not* like what I have to say. Thank you, and have a good day." Closing the door, I leaned up against it, listening for the sound of their car doors to close and their engine to start. Good, they were gone, but would they return?

Two calls were made that evening: one to Mark and one to Richard Haskins. Up until this point, Mark had continued to deny profusely that he was the whistleblower. *How could that be?* I wondered. It had to be him, but because he was insistent, I believed him. I began to wonder about other possibilities. Perhaps it was Stephen? It didn't matter. The truth was out and that was the important factor. As suspected, Mark hadn't spoken to this firm and they were tossing his name around like they were working with him. My suspicions were correct. Richard Haskins provided me with the answer to a question that was a major concern to me: *Do I have to testify again?* He made it clear that he was in no way telling me what to do and that legally, he couldn't.

I didn't want him to tell me what to do. I just needed to understand if I could be subpoenaed by UWP, and would that legal summons require me to take the stand again? I was told "yes." Damn! There was a possibility that this wasn't over yet.

From all appearances, this case was just getting started. I sat down, replaying various scenarios concerning the case. One name stood out. What made them jump on the Swannee hunt? I suspected Audrey had told them I was at the courthouse. When I shared this bit of information with Mr. Haskins, he paused. He asked me to repeat what I had just said.

"I said I encountered a former manager the day I testified."

"Who?" he almost shouted.

"Audrey Sims, a manager from Harborview." Sounding shocked, he demanded to know what she was doing in the courthouse. I assumed he knew and suddenly I panicked.

"No, I had no idea. Something funny is going on here, and I have to check into this. Thank you for bringing this to my attention." Mr. Haskins promised to get back to me once he knew more.

Hanging up the telephone, I allowed my hand to rest on the receiver. Things must really be heating up. People were stooping to deceptive tactics to retrieve information. I vowed to be careful what I said and to whom I now spoke about the case.

Several days later, a newspaper article concerning the investigation made me questions my trust in Mark. There, in bold, black letters, the article declared the whistleblower was "33-year-old Mark Erickson of Seattle." I was flabbergasted. My friend had lied to me. My longtime buddy was the whistle-blower!

UWP wants You

Additional pressure entered my home when I received a surprise call from another investigative firm, retained on behalf of UWP, for assistance in their criminal investigation charges. Vicki Lane, a smooth-talking female, attempted several times to convince me to share information regarding the company. She wanted to know if I would be willing to talk about what I had witnessed at the company. I was beginning to sound like a broken record. I had reached my level of intolerance. This was not something I chose to do; I wasn't going to do it unless forced. I had resigned from UWP years ago, and I wanted nothing more to do with them. During the time I had desperately searched for an avenue to voice problems within the company, management didn't want to hear it. Now I was a hot commodity during this investigation.

Taking a notepad from my desk drawer, I listed concerns I wanted to investigate and additional questions I needed to have answered. The ringing of the telephone interrupted my thought, and for a moment I hesitated before answering it. Lately, there had been so many surprises, I wondered what awaited me on the other end of the telephone. Another surprise—it was Mark Erickson!

Mark was responding to a message I had left on his answering machine. I waited as we said our usual greetings before I said anything more. I felt angry. I had repeatedly asked him if he was the mystery whistleblower, only to be met by firm and insistent bellowing "not me," comment. Now I felt foolish for having believed him.

Mark began to speak, his voice cracking slightly as he did.

"Swannee?"

"Yes," I said dryly on the other end of the telephone. I didn't attempt to hide my slight irritation. "I saw your name in the *Seattle Times*, and it says you are the whistleblower. Is it true?" I pressed, needing him to admit it.

Pausing momentarily he blurted, "Yes, it is me."

"*Why did you lie to me?*" I questioned, sounding more like a hurt girlfriend than his longtime buddy. I needed to understand. This wasn't like him. He briefly explained that he was working with the FBI and wasn't at liberty to discuss any issues that had to do with the case. He couldn't tell anyone the truth, and that included me. Explaining that he didn't want to lie and hoped I understood, I sat back on the other end of the telephone, allowing his words to digest. I didn't like his deception, but it was understandable. This was just the way things were going to have to be for now.

"If opening your mouth and telling anything about this case would affect the outcome, I am glad you kept specifics to yourself. I don't want anything to halt the truth from being revealed," I offered. Sounding relieved by my words, our conversation changed to more lighthearted events. That night was one of the first nights I was able to relax since I had testified before the grand jury. With emotions released, I convinced myself it would all soon be over, but there was another major obstacle coming to my front door.

A Plea for John

Ding Dong, Ding Dong, Ding Dong! It was the middle of the week and I was tired from staying up too late the previous night with my daughter. Making my way towards the front door, I mustered up enough energy to apply a friendly smile on my face.

"Who's visiting us today, little one?" I asked, snuggling her close as I opened the door. A gentleman who appeared to be in his early forties stood poised on my doorstep. He spoke quickly, and in a matter of minutes had introduced himself as Louis Barnes, the attorney representing John Reed. I didn't recognize his name and his words were puzzling.

"I thought Preston, Gates, and Ellis represented John," I frowned, growing suspicious of his presence. He willingly clarified things explaining that Preston, Gates, and Ellis were representing the organization, but John and Paul had hired their own attorneys.

"They must feel like they need some major protection," I teased. His look showed that he was unappreciative of my joke at the moment. *What does he want from me?*

"John needs your help," he stated. I almost laughed. Shifting the weight of my daughter in my arms, I continued the conversation, but I made it obvious by my fixated stance that our talk would be limited to the doorway. Seemingly unaffected by this, he explained that John was facing numerous charges and had mentioned that he knew my mother and me well. My temper flared, but I did my best to conceal it. How dare he try to use the friendship element now, when he was feeling cornered?

"Yes, he knows my mother, but what does that have to do with me now?" I asked. Apparently John had assumed I would be willing to come and speak on his behalf.

I wondered what they thought I could say that would prove beneficial to John. My curiosity about the extreme they were willing to go had peaked. The subject of John's heart troubles was brought up. This was a low blow, and I stressed how worried about John we all had been on many occasions during my employment with UWP.

"Are you aware that he has lost a son from illness?" Louis Barnes questioned.

"I am *very* aware. I knew his son. I was saddened, remembering the pain of John's loss."

"Well, John should no longer have to deal with this sort of stress at his age. The trial has been difficult. The only thing he should be thinking about is his retirement. He thought you would be willing to come and speak about his character. Talk about your friendship and explain that Janine Turner pressed you all to put documentation in the files adding pressure..." I stood there, unable to believe my ears. This was symbolic of a desperate man.

My daughter cooed softly. I pulled her closer, gaining strength from knowing that I was her mother and about to make the right decision.

"Let me tell you something," I began. "John is a nice man, so what I am about to say has nothing to do with him as a person, but there were a lot of things—illegal things—going on in the company that were brought to his attention. He refused to do anything then. It was his job. His responsibility. He didn't want to hear it. In fact, he turned the other cheek when I approached him. Now that he is in trouble, he is asking for my help? Where was he when I almost lost my first child because of all the stress the company placed me under? He didn't care about me then, and I don't care now. I am not crazy about Janine. She did a lot of unforgivable things to many people, but I know she didn't do *all* of these things herself. I refuse to go somewhere and say that she did. I can't do that. So, sir, I cannot help John Reed. I'm sorry. John still thinks I am that young girl he hired, but I am not. I won't do this. I just couldn't live with myself. How I feel at the end of the day when I look in the mirror is more important than anything right now. Now, I need to ask you to please leave."

Hesitantly accepting my response, he offered to leave his telephone number in case I changed my mind.

"Don't bother. I won't," I replied. As I watched him descend the stairs from my home, I closed my front door and leaned against it. My eyes shut tightly. Today I was proud. Proud of the woman I had become.

Going Down, One by One

The criminal investigation of University of Washington Physicians splashed across the front pages of the newspapers like a flood. The media was everywhere, and then there was silence. *All over?* I wondered. They'll never admit the truth, or so I thought, but then there was a resurgence of the case. Despite claiming his intent wasn't to commit fraud, prominent neurosurgeon Dr. Richard Winn admitted to lying to investigators who had investigated Medicare and Medicaid overbilling. Forced to sever all ties with the University Hospital, Winn was placed on probation and agreed to repay $500,000 to Medicare and Medicaid for these over billings. He served 1000 hours of community service, which he chose to do in Nepal. Mount Sinai medical school in New York recently hired Dr. Winn.

Dr. William Couser, chief of the UW medical school's Nephrology division, resigned in February 2002 after more than 20 years in that position. In March 2003, Dr. Couser pleaded guilty to one count of submitting a fraudulent health care bill. He was placed on probation and ordered to pay $100,000 for overbillings.

After 17 years as UWP President, "Paul Petersen" silently resigned his position in November 2001, as federal investigators intensified their inquiry. Mr. Petersen currently works in business development for the school of medicine.

"John Reed" retired his position as UWP Vice President.

Arthur Fontaine, the head of interventional radiology resigned from University Hospital. Group Health Cooperative now employs him.

To settle the federal lawsuit alleging massive overbillings, the University of Washington has agreed to pay $35 million dollars. Whistleblower Mark Erickson is expected to receive approximately 7.25 million for his efforts.

My last conversation with Mark summed up everything. "They are going down one by one, Swannee." I couldn't agree more.

Looking back through the years at all that has happened because of this case, I realize it has had a major impact on my life. Through the events I have experienced, I have learned strength, dedication, forgiveness, and the importance of maintaining one's integrity at all costs. Reliving these circumstances by writing this book has given me a sense of freedom I had never experienced previously. I have learned more about myself as a woman and what type of individual I want to represent in society. It is my hope that by sharing this experience I can touch another individual that may currently be in a similar situation or that may encounter one in the future. Perhaps they will learn that they are not alone and discover often the lone voice is the one that is the most powerful.

Resource Articles-University Physicians Scandal

Smith, Carol. (2002, February 22). Neurosurgery Dept. head told to step down at UW. *Seattle Post Intelligencer.* pp. A1, A13

Smith, Carol. (2002, May 4). Support voiced for UW doctor in fraud inquiry. *Seattle Post Intelligencer.* pp. A1, A5

Smith, Carol. (2002, July 27). UW reaches settlement with convicted brain surgeon. *Seattle Post Intelligencer.* pp. B1

Shukovsky, Paul. Smith, Carol. (2003, March 27). Second UW physician pleads guilty to fraud. *Seattle Post Intelligencer.* pp. A1, A10

Skolnik, Sam. Smith, Carol. (2003, May 1). Key Phase of UW inquiry ends. *Seattle Post Intelligencer.* pp. B1, B8

Smith, Carol. (2003, September 26). UW professor sentenced for role in billing case. *Seattle Post Intelligencer.* pp. B2

Militech, Steve. (2004, January 14). Penalty in UW billing scandal reportedly tops $30 million. *The Seattle Times.* pp. A1, A13

Anderson, Rick. (2004, January 21–27). Postmortem of a Scandal. *Seattle Weekly.* pp A1

Ellison, Jake. (2004, May 1). $35 million later, UW says it didn't cheat. *Seattle Post Intelligencer.* pp. A1, A8

Excerpts

These excerpts have been collected and are being shared as an educational service to benefit readers interested in the University of Washington billing scandal. Presented materials have all been made available to the public via local newspaper publications.

1. "Eminent Surgeon sentenced in billing scandal"
   by Carol Smith

   copyright October 29, 2002
   Washington: *Seattle Post Intelligencer*
   pp. A1, A9

   "Dr. Winn will be an example to others who may have previously believed that their pre-eminence as physicians will shield them from prosecution. Dr. Winn will further be an example to physicians at teaching hospitals who may have otherwise believed that teaching-physician issues would be pursued only as civil matters against their parent institutions."
   U.S. Attorney Susan Loitz

2. "$35 million later, UW says it didn't cheat"
   by Jake Ellison

   copyright May 1, 2004
   Washington: *Seattle Times*
   pp. A1, A8

   "Every single one of the allegations is false."
   UW attorney David Robbins

"It's obvious they were essentially a criminal enterprise."
Referring to the UW Medical Center
San Francisco lawyer, Stephen Meagher

3. "Whistle-blowers say Medicare fraud at the University of Washington was everyday business"
    by Rick Anderson

    copyright June 9–15, 2004
    Washington: *Seattle Weekly*
    pp. 1, 22–27

    "I believe that there are many more doctors in many departments who could have found themselves facing criminal charges."
    Whistle-blower, Mark Erickson

    "I don't know how anyone at the top couldn't know this had gone on."
    Former UWP employee, Swannee Rivers

    "Our physicians and personnel in the practice plans were working very hard to comply with the complicated billing regulations."
    Dean of the UW School of Medicine, Paul Ramsey

4. "UW billing scandal: Did dean do enough?"
    Sharon Chan and Steve Miletich

    copyright June 8, 2004
    Washington: *Seattle Times*
    pp. A1, A13

    "My concern, and the danger I see to the University is that signing and billing for care or supervision (the doctor) has not actually provided probably constituted Medicare and/or insurance fraud."
    Former UW Anesthesiologist, Bruce Spiess

    "That's ridiculous. That's bogus. They're lying about that—gotta be."
    (Comments about UW's lack of knowledge regarding billing issues.)
    UW Physician in departments, Neuroradiology and Neurosurgery, Joe Eskridge

"I do not trust them in the slightest in terms of what they do in…investigations and taking appropriate actions." (Reference to UW criticisms during the billing investigation.)
UW Pediatrics Professor, Warren Guntheroth

"We must accept responsibility—and that, of course, includes me—for improving the compliance program, for the fact that too many errors were made."
Dean of the UW School of Medicine, Paul Ramsey

Valuable Resources in the fight against Medical Fraud

http://www.falseclaimscase.com/

http://www.atg.wa.gov/

http://www.aarp.org/bulletin/medicare/?OVRAW=medicare&
OVKEY=medicare&OVMTC=standard

http://www.aarp.org/consumerprotect/

http://www.wccfighter.com/inthenews.cfm

http://www.hum.wa.gov/

http://www.leg.wa.gov/RCW/index.cfm?fuseaction=chapterdigest&
chapter=42.40

http://www.sao.wa.gov/

0-595-32008-2